T0098765

Mind over Bladder is a tour de force which will benefit all women. As half of all women are affected by incontinence during their lifetime, education about diagnosis and therapy for all is invaluable. The book's authors are a dynamic team of an internationally known authority on pelvic floor disorders and medical education (Jill Rabin) ; an accomplished author who has successfully navigated diagnosis and therapy as a patient (Gail Stein) , and a skilled and sensitive physician and surgeon (Danielle O'Shaughnessy). This trio provides state-of-the-art information in an easy-to-understand format that will greatly enhance understanding of the causes of incontinence and the various options for treatment. Following the adage that 'knowledge is power', readers will come away after reading this book greatly empowered! I strongly recommend this book to all, as it will enhance quality of life for women and their partners throughout the world.

Frank A. Chervenak, MD, MMM
Chair, Obstetrics & Gynecology
Lenox Hill Hospital
Chair, Obstetrics & Gynecology
Associate Dean for International Medicine
Zucker School of Medicine at Hofstra/ Northwell

Mind Over Bladder is a masterful and comprehensive guide for all those living with pelvic support and bladder issues. Accessibly written in a conversational tone, various causes and methods of evaluation are described, as well as a myriad menu of treatments for this common condition. The authors are a true 'Dream Team' with Dr. Rabin (an expert on pelvic floor disorders and incontinence), Dr. O'Shaughnessy (a gifted pelvic surgeon and physician) and Ms. Stein (a seasoned author and patient). This trio's extraordinary combined experience and talent shine a beacon of light on this subject and will most certainly give their readers the power not only of information, but of knowledge.

Michael Nimaroff, MD, MBA
Senior Vice President Executive Director Ob/Gyn Services
Northwell Health

Mind Over Bladder is a wonderful resource for women everywhere. Beautifully co-written with seasoned author Gail Stein, it provides readers with a comprehensive review of pelvic floor disorders, real-life problems unique to women, and a guide to practical solutions. The book is instrumental in accomplishing the Urogynecologic community's aspirations of removing the taboo about discussing often embarrassing, inelegant conditions while proactively educating readers on evaluation and management options for the various pelvic floor disorders. Dr. Rabin, a nationally-renowned clinical expert in the diagnosis and medical management of pelvic floor disorders, and Dr. O'Shaughnessy, a skilled surgeon whose specialty is performing minimally invasive surgical procedures, have combined their talents and experiences treating numerous women with pelvic floor disorders to write *Mind Over Bladder*, a book that will empower women to significantly improve their quality of life and live it to its fullest potential. BRAVO!

Harvey Winkler MD, MBA, FACOG
System Chief, FPMRS: Urogynecology
Professor, Dept of OB/GYN
Donald and Barbara Zucker School of Medicine at Hofstra/Northwell
Program Director, FPM&RS Fellowship

Mind Over Bladder

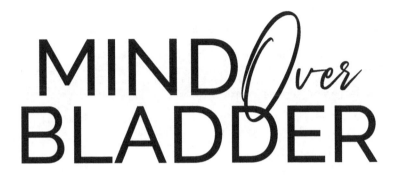

MIND Over BLADDER

A Step-by-Step Guide to Achieving Continence

JILL MAURA RABIN, M.D.
GAIL STEIN

with Danielle O'Shaughnessy, M.D.

NEW YORK

LONDON • NASHVILLE • MELBOURNE • VANCOUVER

Mind Over Bladder

A Step-by-Step Guide to Achieving Continence

Published in New York, New York, by Morgan James Publishing. Morgan James is a trademark of Morgan James, LLC. www.MorganJamesPublishing.com

ISBN 9781631950100 paperback
ISBN 9781631950117 eBook
Library of Congress Control Number: 2020931403

Cover Design by:
Christopher Kirk
www.GFSstudio.com

Interior Design by:
Chris Treccani
www.3dogcreative.net

Back cover graphic by:
Alice H. Brody

Cover design concept by:
Cynthia Busic-Snyder

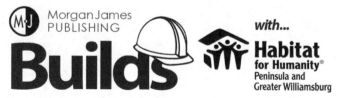

Morgan James is a proud partner of Habitat for Humanity Peninsula and Greater Williamsburg. Partners in building since 2006.

Get involved today! Visit
MorganJamesPublishing.com/giving-back

This book is dedicated to my family: to Bobbie and Aaron for their unwavering support, humor, and love and to Dr. Gertie F. Marx, my treasured mentor and "The Mother of Obstetric Anesthesiology."
J.M.R.

This book is dedicated to my husband, Douglas, for his love and patience; to my children, Eric and Michael, for their encouragement and support; and to the late Barbara Olen, for her wisdom and guidance.
G.S.

Table of Contents

Foreword

Dr. Marvin Terry Grody

When I first met her, Jill Maura Rabin was an obstetrician-gynecologist with a passionate interest in women's health. Having devoted my entire professional career to women's health, one of my primary objectives as instructor and mentor to a future generation of physicians was to impart to them a sense of what a special privilege and responsibility it is to attack the problems that uniquely afflict women and can seriously impair their quality of life. It was clear to me at once that this eager, enthusiastic, and creative practitioner possessed all the personal and professional characteristics qualifying her to bear that responsibility and to share the privilege of caring for women.

Dr. Rabin's subsequent career proved the accuracy of my first impression. Now a nationally recognized authority in urogynecology and female pelvic medicine, she has acquired vast experience with chronic incontinence, one of the principal problems disrupting the quality of women's lives today. Concentrating her efforts on this important specialty, Dr. Rabin has become a leading expert in the management of this embarrassing and debilitating condition that afflicts millions of women across the nation.

With that background, and embellished by extensive clinical research, she has compiled, for the benefit of women everywhere, this admirable volume, unparalleled in scope and clarity, which demystifies a frightening medical problem and thoroughly acquaints the reader with all the currently available therapies. Wisely, Dr. Rabin has divided her topic into four distinct parts, describing each simply and clearly. First, she describes, verbally and pictorially, the various female body parts and mechanisms involved in urination. Next, she details each of the principal incontinence conditions that patients present. Then, she leads the reader through the wide range of neuromuscular, medical, and surgical therapies that currently are available. Last, she explains how and where to seek appropriate advice and care. Everything is offered in language any patient can understand. She intermittently employs the unique and effective literary device of presenting from the first person to enhance readers' comfort.

Dr. Rabin's publication is truly a godsend in its potential to help women beleaguered by chronic incontinence find the way to a much-improved quality of life. Simply put, with Dr. Rabin's invaluable guidance, chronically incontinent women can finally look down and proclaim, "Good-bye, wet pants!"

Marvin H. Terry Grody, MD
Emeritus Professor of Obstetrics and Gynecology,
Robert Wood Johnson Medical School
December 2007

Acknowledgments

To Dr. Gertie F. Marx, the "Mother of Obstetric Anesthesia," my mentor and "medical mother" for her endless, loving advice.

To Dr. George J. Segall, my beloved uncle and gifted diagnostician, who taught by example that the secret in the care of the patient is the caring for the patient.

To my entire family for being there always, with very great love. Especially to my partner, Bobbie, and to my son Aaron, the lights of my life. To my father, the honorable Gilbert Rabin, and my mother, Zita, for teaching me strength and bravery by example, for their love, and for the music. To my loving brother and sister, Corey and Marni, their spouses (really like another sister and brother, Nancy and Thomas), and the children, of course: Erick, Casey, and Abe. To my mother-in-law, Frances (my "other mother"), my loving brother and sister-in-law, Charles and Leanne, and to my niece and gifted physician, Dr. EmmaKate Friedlander.

To Dr. Phyllis Shaw and Dr. Susan Kaiser, for their unwavering belief in me, their friendship, and their meticulous review of the manuscript.

To Ms. Alice H. Brody for her steadfast support, critical editing skills, and a cover design from heaven.

To my friend and colleague for a lifetime, the late Dr. Marvin Terry Grody, for his decades of tireless, loving encouragement and faith in me.

To Marilyn Freedman and Elise Stettner, two of the most gifted pelvic floor physical therapists I have ever known, for their generosity, expertise, and friendship.

To my talented urogynecologic colleague, Dr. Danielle O'Shaughnessy, for her enormous contribution to this revised edition.

To my co-author, Gail Stein. I truly could not do better.

And above all, to my patients and their families. I am honored and humbled by the privilege of caring for and about you. May it continue for many more years.

Jill Maura Rabin, M.D.

Preface

If Not Now, When?

Urinary Incontinence (UI), as defined by the International Continence Society, is "the complaint of any involuntary leakage of urine."[1]

Ten years ago, when this book was first published, I said I would retire when adult women no longer needed diapers. Clearly, this has not yet happened and may take a while longer. Retirement is not on the horizon (nor in my lexicon). Luckily, I am patient (the use of this word to refer to a person receiving medical treatment must not be an etymologic accident, since patients spend so much of their time waiting). Although there are solid, scientific reasons why the continence we learned so well as children may occasionally or even frequently elude us as we get older, as you read this book you will see that urinary incontinence is not an inevitable part of aging. Furthermore, it is not shameful, and when already present, it is treatable in almost every situation. Having said this, millions of women worldwide have experienced urinary incontinence.[2] This is due to several factors: the fact that women's urethras are shorter than men's, at about four centimeters (less than two inches), the changes to pelvic organs and tissues associated with childbirth, and menopause, to name just a few.

The question remains: Why a revised version of *Mind Over Bladder*? Women's anatomy has not changed and there is no substitute for finding a good doctor to

---

1   "What is incontinence?" National Association for Continence Web site (www.NAFC.org). 2006.

2   Ibid.

talk to (your primary doctor, gynecologist, urogynecologist, or urologist) about incontinence. Taking a complete medical history and the need for a full physical exam hasn't changed, nor has the need for a solid diagnostic workup been altered. The answer is very simple and straightforward: our treatment alternatives have greatly improved and, therefore, our patients can expect better outcomes. This newer edition of our book includes all the latest treatment options for each type of incontinence (including the newer, minimally invasive surgeries and newer techniques to quiet an overactive bladder without medication).

When you're ready to address your incontinence head-on, there is no substitute for a thorough diagnostic workup. This starts with a full medical history shared with a physician (or other qualified healthcare provider) whom you trust and who will listen carefully and seriously to your concerns. Explain exactly to him or her in detail how the loss of bladder control is affecting your life physically, socially, and emotionally. Since this issue may have started for you months, or even years ago, and since much "water has passed under the bridge" (pun intended), you might want to write down your questions and concerns ahead of time so you don't miss any important details.

Once a diagnosis has been firmly established, you and your healthcare partner can discuss the various treatment options open to you. Often, in formulating your long-term treatment plan, several options may be chosen and used either simultaneously or sequentially in order to maximize your continence margin (the combination of physical factors that keep you dry at any given point) over the course of your life. Each person's continence margin varies at different times in life. Generally, our margin is wider when we are young, and it may take many factors being "out of sync" to make us lose urine. As we age, our continence margin may be narrower, and a simple urinary tract infection may push us, possibly only temporarily, into the "leakage zone." Nevertheless, it is useful to think of continence as a zone we want to try and remain in as much as possible during the course of our lives and not necessarily as a yes or no, or black and white (or, in this case, yellow or white) issue.

A word about absorbent products (diapers and pads) is in order here. They are, overall, very useful, and their rightful place in the medicines, equipment, and techniques available to a medical practitioner should not be underestimated.

Having said this, I believe that these products work best when utilized as part of the overall plan and not viewed as a treatment, since pads and diapers do not treat urinary incontinence.

Urinary incontinence plagues over half of all nursing home residents and is one of the most common reasons that women enter long-term care and nursing facilities.[3] In the process of losing control of their bladders, they often lose control of their lives as well. Much has been written about the depression associated with untreated incontinence and how lives are negatively affected through the social isolation, emotional turmoil, and physical debilitation that this condition brings. Do not despair! Effective treatments to improve incontinence are currently available, and newer, better treatments are continually being developed while older ones are refined.

Billions of taxpayer dollars—the current estimate is now over thirty billion—are spent on urinary incontinence each year. This money primarily funds the routine care associated with incontinence (such as diapers, skin breakdown care, home health aides) and some of the inadvertent consequences that may be associated with incontinence (e.g., treatment of a hip fracture resulting from a fall on a puddle of leaked urine). In comparison, little money is spent on diagnosis and treatment of this debilitating condition. We all must help to spread the word and work together if we are ever going to make a significant difference.[4]

It is estimated that even today, after all this time, fewer than half of incontinent women share their bladder control issues with their healthcare provider.[5]

It is high time for urinary incontinence to "come out of the water closet." The gestation period of our original book was approximately twelve times the normal nine months, or about nine years! A colleague first proposed the idea to write a

3   Abrams P, Cardozo L, Fall M., et al. 2002. The standardization of terminology of lower urinary tract function: report from the standardization sub-committee of the International Continence Society. Am J Obstet Gynecol 187:116–26.
4   Urinary Incontinence in Adults: Clinical Practice Guideline. AHCPR Pub. No. 92-0038. Rockville, MD: Agency for Healthcare Policy and Research, Public Health Service, U.S. Department of Health and Human Services. March, 1992. Also cited from Thomas TM, Plymat KR, Blannin J, & Meade TW. 1980. Prevalence of urinary incontinence. British Medical J 281(6250):1243–1245.
5   Urinary Incontinence in Adults: Clinical Practice Guideline. AHCPR Pub. No. 92-0038. Rockville, MD: Agency for Healthcare Policy and Research, Public Health Service, U.S. Department of Health and Human Services. March, 1992.

book of this nature in the late 1980s. At that time, at the annual meeting of the American Urogynecologic Society, we were two of the first half-dozen or so female members. Over the next ten years, this colleague's enthusiasm about such a book was echoed by countless patients I had the privilege of helping with their bladder problems, along with the concerns of their spouses, partners, and families. For as I am sure you understand by now, urinary incontinence is a condition that affects not only patients, but whole families and our entire society. This book focuses on the patient, and it is written, for the most part, in and with the voices of my patients. This journey to continence will reassure you that you're not alone in what you're experiencing. All attention is focused "front and center" on the ones whose lives are touched personally by this condition. This revised edition represents a journey that began nearly two decades ago. Certainly, as our understanding of incontinence improves, we can offer our patients better and more effective treatments. Although we still have a long way to go, for now, this journey continues thanks to my colleagues, teachers, and patients: my "medical family."

Now is the time to take charge of your condition, in order to have control over your bladder for life. This book is for all of you—all of us—who know the location of each bathroom in every mall and public place, who spend hours each week doing countless loads of laundry, and whose lives are ruled by their bladders. I believe in "mind over bladder." And at this moment in our history, when we finally know that 'women are not simply small men,' when gender-based research is at the forefront of medical science, the time for us truly is now. If not now, when?

Jill Maura Rabin, MD

Introduction

So You've Finally Had Enough

What's in it for you?

You've just picked up this book, and you're giving it a quick once-over, trying to decide whether or not to purchase it. Here are five compelling reasons why you should grab this copy and read it from cover to cover:

1. It's honest, direct, and to the point.
2. It's co-authored by an understanding, sympathetic expert in gynecology and urology and by a completely satisfied, virtually cured patient.
3. You can understand what's being said because we've eliminated unnecessary medical mumbo jumbo.
4. It includes the latest, up-to-the-minute information available on this topic.
5. The approach is user-friendly.

Recent studies indicate that as many as 50 percent of all women are affected by incontinence. Undoubtedly this is an underestimate, since most women are just too embarrassed to seek help. You don't have to be one of them.[6]

This book seeks to educate women of all ages about the many causes of incontinence and the variety of treatment options available. In chapter 1, we

---

6   Li Y, Cai X, Glance LG, Mukamel DB. 2007. Gender differences in healthcare-seeking behavior for urinary incontinence and the impact of socioeconomic status: a study of the Medicare managed care population. Med Care. Nov; 45(11):1116–22.

define incontinence and explain some of the primary factors that can cause it. We also discuss some of the myths and legends surrounding incontinence.

Chapter 2 explores the female urinary tract and explains the anatomical components of this complex system. We discuss how the brain and spinal cord coordinate the muscles and organs that regulate the flow of urine.

Chapter 3 addresses the conditions and causes of incontinence in women. We discuss risk factors, chemicals that stimulate the urge to urinate, and how natural events in the body, such as pregnancy and menopause, can affect incontinence.

In chapter 4, we discuss the process of selecting a physician to treat your incontinence, as well as what to expect from the initial round of tests that will be performed. You'll review a list of questions to ask potential physicians and learn what questions you should expect from your physician.

Stress incontinence is one of the most common diagnoses that incontinent women receive, so we devote chapter 5 to a discussion of the definition, triggers, sources, and results of stress incontinence. We differentiate between minimal, moderate, and severe forms of the condition and discuss a variety of treatment options.

The second most common form of incontinence is urge incontinence, the frequent sensation that urination is imminent and cannot be postponed for long. And though it is rare that an actual cause can be determined for urge incontinence, in chapter 6 we discuss likely sources that exacerbate the condition and some potential treatments.

Aside from the two common forms of incontinence, there are other types of urinary incontinence, which we review in chapter 7. These conditions vary widely in their symptoms and preferred methods of treatment.

At the other end of the spectrum from incontinence is urinary retention, a condition in which the bladder does not empty properly. In chapter 8, we examine the symptoms, likely causes, and remedies for this condition.

More than 5.5 million Americans suffer from fecal incontinence, so we devote chapter 9 to a frank discussion of this condition.[7] Because physicians' methods for diagnosing this ailment obviously differ from the tests we've discussed for

7 Whitehead WE, Palsson OS, Simre M. Treating fecal incontinence: an unmet need in primary care medicine. *North Carolina Medical Journal.* 2016;77(3):211-215.

urinary incontinence, we'll cover the procedures and examinations you could expect to undergo during a preliminary diagnosis. Because some symptoms of fecal incontinence can be managed with dietary adjustments, we review changes you can easily make with the approval of your physician.

Because of the complications and risks inherent in surgery, it's usually a good idea to explore non-surgical treatments for incontinence first. So chapter 10 explores the wide variety of non-surgical treatment options for urinary incontinence. Physical therapy, behavior modification, voiding diaries, bladder training, Kegel exercises, vaginal cones and weights, biofeedback devices, pessaries, intravaginal devices, acupuncture, and forms of medication are all safe and effective treatments for incontinence, and we discuss them in turn.

Unfortunately, despite any number of safer treatments considered or tried, patients must sometimes undergo surgery to achieve the control over incontinence they desire; we discuss such conditions in chapter 11. Surgery for incontinence is almost always an elective treatment option, though it is a medical necessity in rare circumstances. We review some of the different forms of surgical treatment and the risks and outcomes that surgical patients can expect.

Chapter 12 considers some naturally occurring conditions that lend themselves to incontinence, such as pregnancy, menopause, and illnesses such as interstitial cystitis, multiple sclerosis, and Parkinson's disease. We also discuss the implications of birth defects like spina bifida and other medical conditions like strokes and Alzheimer's.

Throughout this book, we employ a number of elements to draw your attention to topics of interest. One of the most common of these is **Tech Terms,** which defines important terminology surrounding incontinence. **Q&A** boxes complement frequently asked questions about incontinence with straight-talk answers. **Dos and Don'ts** offer practical tips for dealing with situations surrounding the management and treatment of incontinence. In the **Believe It or Not** boxes, my patients recount some of their more dramatic experiences with incontinence; they make you laugh or cry, and they'll definitely assure you that you're not alone in what you're experiencing. Finally, each chapter concludes with **The Wrap-Up**, a summary of the most important points to remember.

Now that we've explained the intent of our book, we encourage you to turn the page and begin what we hope will be an educational and, ultimately, healing experience.

Why Read This Book?

Chapter Highlights

- Why Us?
- Staggering Statistics
- Myths and Legends
- Developing a Strategy: "Never Say Die"
- What We Offer
- The Wrap-Up

Incontinence! Face it, ladies. Doesn't the sound of that word make you want to cringe? How about run and hide? If your answer is a resounding "Yes!" followed by a sense of panic, and perhaps even tears, there's good news! Your fears are unfounded, and it can be possible for you to be "high and dry" forever.

TECH TERMS

Urinary Incontinence (UI), as defined by the International Continence Society, is "the complaint of any involuntary leakage of urine."[8]

---
8   Op. cit. "What is Incontinence?"

Why Us?

Girls, the sad but true fact is that incontinence primarily strikes women. Whoever said that life is fair? So why does this happen to us? Unfortunately, our pelvic anatomy works against us.

DOS AND DON'TS

Do feel free to discuss any bladder control or incontinence problems you may experience with a qualified professional. You aren't alone, and no one is going to make fun of you.

Women are susceptible to bladder infections, also known as urinary tract infections (UTIs) or cystitis.

Have you ever had one? If so, you know that the pain, burning, and urinary frequency are symptoms you'd like to avoid at all costs. Bacteria can easily enter women's bladders because our vagina, urethra, and anus are close together and because our short urethras make it easier for germs to travel where they shouldn't go.

TECH TERMS

Located above the vaginal opening, the **urethra** is a short, narrow tube that carries urine from the bladder out of the body.

We get pregnant. You might expect some leakage during pregnancy as the uterus enlarges and puts increased pressure on the bladder. Why? The bladder and pelvis undergo changes during pregnancy to accommodate the growing fetus and the mother. The bladder may not empty as well because of pressure from the enlarging uterus or fetus, which may lead to an increase in the amount of urine left in the bladder after urinating. This remaining urine may be the perfect environment for bacterial growth, which may cause the increased occurrence of urinary tract infections during pregnancy. There is also an increase in the amount of urine produced by the kidneys. As a result, pregnant women have to urinate more frequently. Several hormones produced during pregnancy (especially estrogen and progesterone) cause relaxation in pelvic tissues and organs, including the bladder and ureters (tubes leading from the kidneys to the bladder). This relaxation is helpful because it allows the pelvis to become more flexible and to make room for that baby; however, it may also lead to incomplete bladder emptying and UTIs. In addition to this, pregnancy and delivery may also cause nerve damage to the pelvic muscles, which may not heal completely and cause subsequent problems.

TECH TERMS

Prolapse is the dropping of the uterus, the bladder, or rectum into the vagina. Prolapse occurs when the uterus protrudes or sags into the vagina.

A woman's first delivery carries the greatest risk of long-term incontinence. Pregnancy and delivery can damage the muscles, nerves, and other structures supporting the pelvis, causing a loss of support of the uterus, bladder, and rectum. If recovery is not complete, incontinence may result, in large part due to prolapse of these organs. Vaginal delivery has been shown to be the single largest predictor of incontinence. There is a statistically significant relationship between the number of vaginal deliveries and the incidence of incontinence: as the number of vaginal deliveries for a woman increases, so does the probable incidence of incontinence.[9]

Deliveries that are performed with the assistance of instruments, such as forceps, carry an even higher risk than normal vaginal deliveries. Caesarean section may minimize some of the effects of incontinence and prolapse.

Menopause is another leading cause of incontinence. Estrogen levels drop during menopause, the muscles and tissues in the pelvis lose strength and support

---

9   Nygaard I, Cruickshank D. 2003. Should all women be offered elective caesarean delivery? Obstet and Gynecol 102:217–219.

due to lower levels of collagen (a supporting protein in the skin), and organs prolapse. Low estrogen levels may also result in atrophy (a thinning of tissues of the body, or type of tissue wasting), which causes the walls of the vagina and bladder to become inflamed and easily damaged. This may cause pelvic soreness and itching. In addition, the urethra may become irritated, which may lead to increased urinary frequency and urinary tract infections.

Staggering Statistics

You are not alone—far from it! Here are some facts and figures about the many people actually affected by incontinence:

- Urinary incontinence affects 200 million people worldwide.[10]
- Of the twenty-five million adult Americans suffering from some form of urinary incontinence, 75 to 80 percent are women.[11]
- Approximately 23 percent of women over the age of sixty experience incontinence.[12]
- One in four women over the age of eighteen experiences episodes of involuntary urine leakage.[13]
- Five percent of children at five years of age have problems with bed-wetting, and 1 to 2 percent continue to have the problem past the age of fifteen.[14]
- Not surprisingly, both the prevalence and the severity of urinary incontinence increases with age.
- On average, women wait six and a half years from the first time they experience symptoms before they obtain a diagnosis for their bladder control problems.[15]

---

10 Ibid,
11 https://www.nafc.org/facts and statistics
12 Ibid.
13 Ibid.
14 Fergusson DM, Horwood LJ, Shannon FT. Factors related to the age of attainment of nocturnal bladder control: an 8-year longitudinal study. Pediatrics 1986; 78:884.
    Bakker E, van Sprundel M, van der Auwera JC, et al. Voiding habits and wetting in a population of 4,332 Belgian schoolchildren aged between 10 and 14 years. Scand J Urol Nephrol 2002; 36:354.
15 Ibid.

- Stress urinary incontinence, the most prevalent form of incontinence among women, affects an estimated fifteen million adult women in the U.S.[16]
- About 17 percent of women and 16 percent of men over the age of eighteen have an overactive bladder (OAB) and an estimated 12.2 million adults have urge incontinence.[17]
- Urinary incontinence is twice as common in women as in men.[18]
- Pregnancy, childbirth, and menopause are the major causes in the increased prevalence of incontinence in women.[19]
- More than 50 percent of women in nursing homes report urinary incontinence.[20]
- Approximately 66 percent of men and women between the ages thirty and seventy have never discussed their bladder health with their doctor.[21]
- Over two-thirds of women don't associate losing urine when coughing or sneezing with a medical disorder or health problem.[22]
- One-third of all women think that loss of bladder control is a natural result of aging.[23]
- Adult diaper sales cost taxpayers approximately eleven billion dollars a year, and this figure only includes products needed for people over sixty-five years of age.[24]
- The typical sufferer of urinary incontinence spends 1,000 to 3,000 dollars annually on absorbent products.[25]
- The cost of urinary incontinence for taxpayers for individuals over sixty-five years of age was over $26.3 billion per year.[26]

---

16 Ibid.
17 Ibid.
18 WomensHealth.gov, Urinary incontinence fact sheet
19 Ibid.
20 Op. cit. "What is Incontinence?"
21 Ibid.
22 Op. cit. "What is Incontinence?"
23 Ibid.
24 Wagner. 1998. Economic Considerations of Overactive Bladder. Urology 51(3)355–361.
25 Culligan PJ, Heit M. 2000. Urinary Incontinence in Women: Evaluation and Management. December 1.
26 Op cit. Wagner.

- Approximately 80 percent of those suffering from urinary incontinence can be helped or completely cured.[27]
- Despite the high success rate in treating incontinence, only one out of every twelve people affected gets help, and once symptoms develop, that person will wait an average of seven years before seeing a healthcare professional.[28]

Myths and Legends

Women don't get help with problems of incontinence because they believe in one or more of these myths:

1. **I'm too young to be incontinent.** Incontinence can occur at any age, even in the very young, and it can be treated and corrected to avoid future problems. Young people can be incontinent for a variety of reasons, including over-exercising, childbirth, or injury. Ten to 80 percent of high-impact elite female athletes report urinary incontinence. [29]

2. **It's just too late for me to fight incontinence.** With proper treatment and a sympathetic and understanding doctor, incontinence may be avoided and treated.

3. **Leaking doesn't make me incontinent.** Any leaking, however little, is a symptom of incontinence. It shows that there's a problem that needs immediate attention.

4. **Incontinence naturally comes with age.** Incontinence isn't caused by age, and most older people manage to stay dry. The aging process, however, can make a woman more likely to experience incontinence.

5. **All I need is a pill or a diaper.** Despite what you might see on TV, neither of these represents a real solution to incontinence. Medicine can cause side effects, and undergarments are frequently uncomfortable. While these treatments temporarily address the symptoms of incontinence, the only long-term solution is to address the problem head-on.

---

27   Op. cit. "What is Incontinence?"
28   Ibid.
29   de Mattos Lourenco, T. R., Matsuoka, P. K., Baracat, E. C., & Haddad, J. M. (2018). Urinary incontinence in female athletes: a systematic review. *International urogynecology journal*, *29*(12), 1757-1763.

6. **Incontinence is untreatable.** This is the biggest myth of all. Below are just some of the options available to you today. They range from totally non-invasive therapies to surgery. Your doctor can tell you what will work best for you.
   - Modifying your behavior
   - Restricting your diet
   - Retraining your bladder
   - Doing Kegels (pelvic muscle exercises)
   - Using biofeedback therapy
   - Taking medication
   - Checking your medications with your doctor, because there are over 300 medications that may cause incontinence
   - Undergoing surgery—either in your doctor's office or in a hospital operating room

BELIEVE IT OR NOT

I first realized that I had a considerable problem when I was a teen-ager and constantly had to carry a sweater or jacket to hide the wet stains I left on the back of my pants. Whenever I laughed, I just couldn't hold back the flow of urine. It felt like a dam had opened and all the water in my body just gushed out. How embarrassing it was to be out with my boyfriend and feel the liquid streaming down my legs and then have to try to cover my accident with any-thing in sight. My most mortifying moment was when I left a huge stain on a friend's pastel blue sofa. I never told anyone how severe the problem was, and it only got worse with age.

Developing a Strategy: "Never Say Die"

Now that you know that there are very real, very practical, very easy options available to you, you can focus on developing a strategy that will allow you to enjoy the freedom of being continent. This book will walk you through what to do:

1. Examine your problem—keep a bladder diary and note the foods you eat.
2. Select a doctor—make sure you choose someone who is a specialist in urodynamics, such as a urogynecologist (an OB/GYN who has specialized training in female urology) or urologist.
3. Get a thorough examination and evaluation.
4. Examine your options.
5. Choose the best course of action for you.
6. Work at achieving your goal.

TECH TERMS

Urodynamics is the study of and a series of tests determining how the bladder, urethra, and pelvic floor muscles function.

What We Offer

Urinary incontinence is as common as heart disease and arthritis, but I'm sure you are much more likely to lean over to a friend in a restaurant and say, "I just had a little chest pain; would you call 911?" or "My arthritis is killing me," rather than, "I just laughed so hard I peed in my pants." You know what I mean. It's time for incontinence to come out of the closet. So ask yourself these questions:

- Does your bladder rule your life?
- Do you know the location of a bathroom everywhere you go (especially when shopping)?
- When you're somewhere new, do you scout out the bathrooms as quickly as possible?
- Do you avoid long trips because you might be too far from a restroom?
- Do you leak when you laugh, cough, sneeze, lift, hear running water, have your keys in the front door?
- Do you have trouble making it to the bathroom?
- Do you run to the bathroom several times an hour?
- Do you have sudden, uncontrollable urges to use a bathroom?
- Do you wake up often during the night?

- Can your incontinence be treated and, in some cases, even cured?

If you answered "yes" to any of these questions, we offer you a book that will give you back your freedom and help you regain control of your bladder and your life without pads, without pills, and perhaps without surgery.

The Wrap-Up

- This book offers an informative, easy-to-understand guide to a problem that's more prevalent than you think.
- You definitely aren't alone, and you certainly shouldn't be embarrassed. If our anatomy is our destiny, we can make it work for us.
- Any woman, young or old, can successfully deal with incontinence.
- The goal of continence can be reached by following a strategy.
- You can regain the freedom and control you want and need.

Why We Stay Dry
(How Our Plumbing Works)

Chapter Highlights

- The Urinary Tract: Your Passageway to Continence
- The Kidneys: Your Filtering System
- The Ureters: Your Transportation System
- The Bladder: Your Storage Tank
- The Urethra: Your Drainage Tube
- The Sphincters: Your Control System
- The Pelvic Floor: Your Support System
- The Brain and the Spinal Cord: Your Command Center
- Way to Go
- The Wrap-Up

I never told a soul, not even my very best friend at the time, Katy. But I'll share my secret with you, because I venture to guess that most of you have had a similar experience. It happened one day after a class in biology in junior high school. I ran home and pulled out my mother's 7x magnifying mirror. Then I dropped my panties and carefully positioned the mirror between my legs so that it caught the perfect angle for optimal viewing in our dim bathroom light. I simply couldn't believe what Mr. Wieser, our seventh-grade biology teacher, had told us: that women had three openings "down there," while guys had only two. I just had to see it for myself. I spent an inordinate amount of time that day examining myself and, lo and behold, the man was right! I finally found what I was looking for. Did anyone else have a similar experience?

TECH TERMS

The **urinary tract** is the passageway through which bodily waste products are filtered and through which urine is produced, stored, and excreted.

The Urinary Tract: Your Passageway to Continence

We remain continent when the organs (kidneys, bladder, brain), tubes (ureters and the urethra), and muscles (sphincter muscles and the pelvic floor muscles), as well as the spinal cord, that comprise and control the urinary tract, function properly. The upper urinary tract consists of the kidneys and the ureters that are attached to them. The bladder and the urethra are in the lower urinary tract. Continence is achieved when the entire urinary system works like a well-tuned motor: when there is normal lower urinary tract support and normal functioning of the sphincter muscles.

The Kidneys: Your Filtering System

Most people have two bean-shaped kidneys, which are located in the back on either side of the spinal cord and are protected by the rib cage and a layer of fat. The kidneys constantly filter the body's blood supply by separating and eliminating toxins and waste products from things that the body needs, such as certain nutrients, in order to maintain homeostasis.

TECH TERMS

Homeostasis refers to the balance of the body's internal environment, e.g., blood pressure, temperature, blood sugar level.

Urine is a combination of about 5 percent of these dissolved waste products (urea, uric acid, and creatinine) and about 95 percent of excess water. The kidneys adjust the composition of urine in order to maintain water balance, electrolyte concentrations, the secretion of certain hormones, and the activation of vitamin D. It doesn't make sense to put the bladder before the ureters, since the ureters transport urine to the bladder.

The Ureters: Your Transportation System

The ureters are narrow, hollow, muscular tubes, approximately nine inches long, that connect the kidneys to the bladder. Each kidney has its own ureter through which urine passes. Urine does not flow in a slow, steady stream along the length of the ureters into the bladder. The walls of the ureters are composed of smooth, involuntary muscles that contract at the rate of anywhere between one and five times per minute and, by means of regular, peristaltic waves and gravity, push urine in spurts of about one and a half teaspoons toward the bladder for storage and for later elimination. You are totally unaware when your ureters are working because they are completely out of your control and are set in motion by electrical impulses inside your brain.

TECH TERMS

Peristalsis refers to waves of muscular contractions that can occur in the ureter as well as in other organs of the body.

The Bladder: Your Storage Tank

Bladder function is very complex. It requires that the front part of the brain (the cerebral cortex), which controls when and where to urinate, coordinates with the back part of the brain (the pons), which allows the bladder, the urethra, and the pelvic muscles to work together effectively and efficiently. Since bladder control depends on many variables, different problems may arise that cause different types of incontinence with different types of remedies. For this reason, it is essential to understand how the bladder works.

TECH TERMS

The **micturition reflex** refers to urination: the relaxation of the sphincter muscles, the contraction of the bladder, the relaxation and opening of the urethra, and the act of voiding.

The bladder, a hollow, muscle-lined sac located in the lower abdomen, has two main roles: to store urine and then later to eliminate it. The ureters enter the bladder at an oblique angle and remain in the bladder wall for about another inch. The ureteral outlet into the bladder remains open only when peristalsis (contraction) is occurring, so that urine doesn't flow back from the bladder to the kidney. As urine enters it, the bladder relaxes, thus allowing it to act as an expandable storage tank, continually accommodating an increasing amount of fluid without a significant increase in internal bladder pressure. When empty, the bladder resembles a deflated balloon. As it fills, however, the bladder continually changes shape until it resembles a pear. The detrusor muscle, located within the bladder wall, expands as urine is stored and contracts when it is eliminated. During storage, urine is held within the bladder by a ring of muscles at the bottom of the bladder (the urethral sphincter), which remains shut and increasingly tightens as the bladder fills. As the bladder fills, signals are sent to receptors in the cerebral cortex of the brain telling it what is occurring, while other inhibitory signals are sent from the brain to prevent premature emptying of the bladder.

The bladder neck is the opening at the bottom of the bladder where it connects to the urethra. The bladder neck is surrounded by muscles that keep it closed so that urine remains in the bladder as it fills and is eliminated only during urination. Urine should only move through the bladder neck to the urethra during voluntary urination, when the bladder muscles contract and the bladder neck muscles relax.

DOS AND DON'TS

Don't try to forcibly hold your urine too long. If you stretch the bladder too much, your muscles may weaken, and you may start to "dribble" as you get older. Beware: this condition is harder to fix than incontinence. Once a muscle is stretched, that's it; there's no way to regain your tone!

TECH TERMS

The **detrusor muscle** makes up the entire outside of the bladder and is responsible for contracting the bladder during urination.

The Urethra: Your Drainage Tube

In women, the urethra is a small, narrow tube measuring about one and a half inches that is located just above the vaginal opening. With a good magnifying mirror and patience, it can be located with the naked eye. Your urethra is the tube that carries urine from the bladder to the outside of your body; in other words, the urethra is all that stands between your bladder and the outside world. During bladder filling, it is closed and sealed so that it is watertight. At the time of urination, the urethra opens completely and the top of the bladder contracts. After urination has occurred, the urethra closes and the bladder relaxes again.

Continence depends on several active and passive properties of the detrusor muscle and the urethra. The detrusor is passive when it is filling and active when it is emptying or undergoing unstable contraction. The urethra is active when it is filling and passive when it is emptying. Normal detrusor function allows bladder filling with little or no change in pressure. Detrusor overactivity is characterized by involuntary detrusor contractions during the filling phase. All systems have to be "go" before you can relieve yourself. If the time and the place aren't right, it just isn't going to happen: I know this firsthand!

BELIEVE IT OR NOT

I am and always have been a party girl, so I never pass up the opportunity to have some fun. Many years ago, I had a summer job in the city and, every Friday, any serious work stopped at noon. On one particular steamy day in July, the drop-dead-gorgeous, extremely eligible company VP took a co-worker and me out for a two-martini (well, maybe it was three, but who's counting!) lunch at a fabulous, posh restaurant to celebrate our upcoming birthdays. Although I unconsciously drooled into my drinks as I stared into Mr. R's cerulean blue eyes, that did nothing to diminish the potency of all I was imbibing. Alas, it was finally time to go, and the forty-five minute-trip home to Flushing on the number seven train was going to be a long one. Naturally, I stopped in the ladies room first and drained my bladder till it was beyond empty.

The ride home was uneventful until I arrived at my stop. Gee, I remarked, I really had to go again, and I was feeling a bit uncomfortable. I still had about a twenty-minute walk, but I was young and I felt confident that I could make it home without a problem. Besides, I absolutely refused to stop in any of those seedy, filthy bathrooms in the fast-food joints I passed—they were disgusting beyond words. Big mistake that was!

By the time I was five blocks away from my destination, as the tears welled up from the excruciating pain I felt, I tried and tried with all my might to let go and just pee in my pants. It just wouldn't happen, despite the fact that I felt as though my bladder was going to burst any second.

I finally made it to my apartment and bolted for the bathroom, where, in fact, it took a few minutes for me to relax and finally do what needed to be done. Ladies, as you can see, the time, the place, and your comfort zone are so important when it comes to bladder control.

The Sphincters: Your Control System

A sphincter is a muscle that surrounds a body opening (the urethra or the anus, for example) and which should unconsciously remain tightly closed.

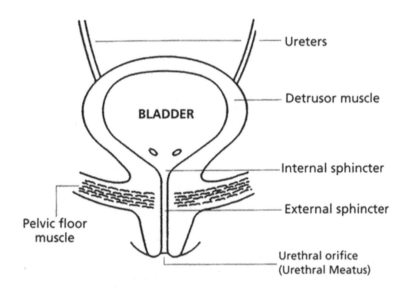

Female Urinary System. Reprinted with permission. *The Urinary Incontinence Sourcebook*. McGraw Hill Education, Copyright 1999.

During urination, sphincters relax and open when messages are relayed from your nerves and your brain to the pelvic floor muscles. Internal and external sphincter muscles control the storage and voiding of urine. The internal sphincter instinctively squeezes the urethra closed. The external sphincter is more under your control for short periods of time and can be squeezed to prevent the leakage of urine when you sneeze, cough, laugh, or do anything that puts additional pressure on your bladder. The internal and external sphincter muscles work in tandem, expanding and contracting as the bladder fills and empties. Nerves automatically relay messages to your muscles ensuring that the sphincters remain closed and that you don't leak.

When enough urine has accumulated in the bladder and it has filled to the point that its internal pressure has increased and its bladder wall has stretched, your nervous system sends a message to your brain, which in turn sends a message to your bladder's detrusor muscle, telling it to relax the internal sphincter muscle. When that happens, the external sphincter muscle becomes tight, and you have a distinct urge to urinate. When you are ready to urinate, you relax your external sphincter, and urine flows.

DOS AND DON'TS

Don't expect to constantly feel the need to urinate. It takes time for the bladder to fill to the point where you will become aware of the increasing volume of urine in it.

The Pelvic Floor: Your Support System

Your pelvic floor muscles are strong, flexible, and voluntary skeletal muscles that you can control and can strengthen or "pump up" through exercise in order to maintain continence. Attached to your pubic bone and to your tailbone (a.k.a. your coccyx), the pelvic floor muscles act as a sling to support and anchor the organs they surround within the abdomen: the uterus, the bladder, and the rectum. Weakness, loss of muscle tone, or damage to the pelvic floor muscles can cause these organs to shift or sag, creating a condition known as pelvic organ prolapse.

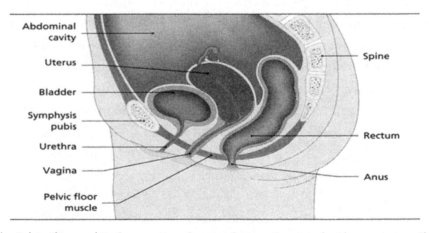

The Pelvic Floor and Its Organs: Your Support System. Reprinted with permission. *The Urinary Incontinence Sourcebook*. McGraw Hill Education, Copyright 1999.

Keep your pelvic floor muscles in excellent shape by doing Kegel exercises. There are two good reasons why:

1. Good pelvic floor muscle tone helps prevent incontinence.
2. A woman can flex her pelvic floor muscles during intercourse to greatly increase her pleasure and to stimulate her partner beyond his expectations.

Here's how to tell that you are doing a Kegel correctly: Insert a tampon into your vagina. Then tug on the string and prevent yourself from removing it. The muscles you feel contracting are your pelvic floor muscles.

Here's a third reason for those of us approaching or in our golden years: as women age and move toward and experience menopause, their estrogen levels drop, thus weakening their pelvic floor muscles. This makes remaining continent problematic for some, so doing Kegels is the way to go!

Your pelvic floor muscles are responsible for contracting at the right time so that you can hold in your urine and for relaxing at the right time so that you can urinate. So, as you can see, keeping them healthy is essential for maintaining continence.

The Brain and the Spinal Cord: Your Command Center

Your brain and your spinal cord serve as the command center for bladder control. They coordinate the bladder, the bladder neck, the urethra, and the pelvic floor muscles. Messages exchanged between the brain and the spinal cord that travel to the body's muscles and organs are responsible for a person's continence or incontinence. When each system involved in bladder control receives and responds appropriately to these messages, continence is achieved. A breakdown in communication, which may be caused by physical or mental conditions, results in incontinence. It's as simple as that.

BELIEVE IT OR NOT

It was 6:00 a.m. and I had just given birth to my first child. He was delivered in his breech position at 12:30 a.m., feet first, and I was sore, exhausted, and groggy from the anesthetic the doctor had slipped into my IV unbeknownst to me. I had been trying to get a little rest when a big, unfriendly, no-nonsense nurse forced me out of my cozy bed and onto the nearby toilet so that she could measure my urine. Little did I know that voiding was such a big deal! There I was, modest me, bathroom door ajar, my hospital gown open and exposing everything to the three other women patients looking on, and this overworked, nasty behemoth, with her hands on hips, ordering me in her harshest voice to "pee already."

I sat there and sat there and pushed and grunted, but absolutely nothing happened; my bashful bladder threatened to do me in. The lady in white got even more annoyed and warned me that if I didn't go soon, I'd fall victim to the agony of catheterization. Anything but that!

I had had enough. I was on the verge of tears when a magnificent, self-preserving thought struck me. I looked Nurse Ratched in the eyes and said in my sweetest voice, "Would you mind please shutting the door?" Luckily for me, she complied, and within a minute, my urine was flowing and a smile returned to my face. As you may well know, you just have to be comfortable for your parts to work properly.

Way To Go

So how is bladder control achieved? The kidneys make urine, which in turn trickles down the ureters. The ureters carry urine to the bladder. The bladder relaxes and fills, and the entire urethra tightens to hold in the urine. The formation of urine in the bladder and its storage in the kidneys are both involuntary processes. When the bladder is full, it sends a message to the brain that it needs to be emptied, and you get the sensation that you have to urinate. If you are continent, the time and the place have to be right—otherwise, your parts just won't work. Self-discipline prevails. If you must hold it in, you will deliberately and voluntarily tighten your pelvic muscles, cross your legs, hold yourself, or do whatever is necessary until the perfect opportunity presents itself. If you wait too long, believe me, you will start to feel pain. Once you find a suitable bathroom, your brain signals your pelvic muscles to relax and your bladder to contract. Voilà: a successful voiding experience!

The Wrap-Up

- Your urinary tract is responsible for your continence or incontinence.
- Your kidneys maintain your body's homeostasis by filtering the blood supply and by separating and eliminating toxins and waste products from those things that the body needs.
- Your ureters transport urine from the kidneys to the bladder.
- Your bladder is responsible for storing and eliminating urine.
- Your urethra carries urine from your bladder to the outside of your body.
- Your sphincters control the storage and voiding of urine.
- Your pelvic floor supports and anchors the organs they surround within the abdomen: the uterus, the bladder, and the rectum.
- Your brain and your spinal cord are responsible for your continence or your lack thereof.

3

Why We Leak

Chapter Highlights
- Let's Get Physical
- Risk Factors for Urinary Incontinence
- Mind Over Matter, Mind Over Bladder
- Time To Go
- The Wrap-Up

I think I must have been incontinent from birth, if that is at all possible. On any given day, from early childhood until the day I got married (I kid you not), the ammonia-like fragrance of dried, stale urine emanated from beneath my bed. That's where I hid my soaked, yellow-stained panties from my mother when I had yet another "accident." My tattletale sister must have suffered from clogged nasal passages, because she never detected the odor of *eau d'urine* when we shared a room as children. My mother must have needed a change in her eyeglass prescription (there was no laser surgery way back then) not to have noticed how discolored my white cotton panties had become.

As a child, I didn't leak. Oh no! Instead, every time I laughed just a little too hard, the dam would burst, and I would wet myself again. I never told a soul, and no one ever surmised what was happening. As you can well imagine, my "accidents" were a very stressful, painful, humiliating part of my childhood.

Let's Get Physical

Don't you ever wonder why can one person hold it in like a camel, for a seemingly endless amount of time, while another person constantly has to go or risk losing control? Urinary frequency and urgency may be caused by a variety of different physical conditions. We leak because of a medical condition or because we are simply doing something wrong. Once our problems are cured or we change our habits, our bladders respond appropriately, and we can once again enjoy continence.

Risk Factors for Urinary Incontinence

So who, exactly, is at risk for developing a problem with incontinence? The list that follows gives the risk factors for any of the varying types of urinary incontinence:

- Gender and Age
- Pelvic Muscle Weakness
- Pregnancy and Childbirth
- Pelvic Surgery
- Menopause
- Medications
- Low Fluid Intake
- High Fluid Intake
- Constipation
- Smoking
- Obesity
- Caffeine
- Food Products (tomatoes, citrus)
- High-Impact Physical Activities
- Urinary Tract/Bladder Infection
- Interstitial Cystitis
- Illnesses and Medical Events
- Anatomic and Neurological Abnormalities

Gender and Age

Urinary incontinence affects more than twenty-five million Americans and twice as many women as men. This is in large part because women have shorter urethras, which measure only about three to five centimeters. In men, the urethra must travel approximately twenty centimeters from the bladder through the prostate gland and then through the penis. In addition to that, the male urethra is better developed, because it is also responsible for preventing the backflow of ejaculate during orgasm. In women over twenty years old, the prevalence of urinary incontinence approaches 20 percent. The prevalence of incontinence increases with age.[30]

Pelvic Muscle Weakness

No matter how active a woman has been during her earlier life, her muscle tone will decrease and her muscles will tend to weaken as she ages. Weak pelvic and abdominal muscles can lead to stress incontinence as well as other forms of incontinence.

BELIEVE IT OR NOT

I was in the throes of perimenopause. The hair on my head was thinning while the hairs on my chin were sprouting. My mood swings knew no bounds, and my sleep pattern was interrupted as I constantly woke up drenched in sweat that flowed non-stop out of every pore of my body. I acquired a pot belly, thirty extra pounds, sagging boobs, pain in my lower back, and increased problems with incontinence. Once a svelte, hot, sexy babe, I now looked like a dowdy, aging matron, and I seemed to spend half my life in the bathroom.

I joined a gym, found a wonderful orthopedist, and went to the best urogynecologist (who, amazingly, accepted my medical insurance) in the world. She, in turn, recommended the most knowl-

---

30   Swenson, C. (2018). Urinary Incontinence: An Inevitable Part of Aging?

edgeable, the most compassionate, and the most competent physical therapist specializing in incontinence to walk the planet. My bladder control assignment, among other things, included doing two to three sets of Kegel exercises per day to strengthen and to improve the tone of my pelvic muscles. At first I did them diligently, without fail, and with remarkable results. But when I felt confident that my incontinence was under control, I admit to you all that I got increasingly lazy and complacent. After a while, I stopped doing the Kegels altogether.

When I went back to the urogynecologist for my yearly checkup, you know what hit the fan. She calmly and patiently explained that my pelvic muscles, like the other muscles in my body, weaken with age and without use. What I had done, by neglecting to exercise, was allow my pelvic floor muscles to atrophy a bit. The doctor explained that if I didn't start doing my Kegels again immediately, and that if I didn't do them regularly and conscientiously, my incontinence would return. My suggestion to you all, even if you aren't experiencing any problems at the moment, is to start doing those Kegels right away and continue doing them forever. There is no downside.

Pregnancy

Pregnancy and childbirth can result in temporary or permanent bladder control problems. During pregnancy, the amount of urine produced by the kidneys increases, resulting in an increase in the frequency of urination. As the fetus grows, the uterus enlarges and puts greater pressure on the bladder, which may lead to leakage (that usually stops after childbirth). About half of all first-time pregnancies result in bladder control problems, especially during the last trimester.[31] Pregnancy can also cause damage to the nerves that control the pelvic muscles. If this damage does not heal, incontinence problems may result.

---

31 Wesnes, S. L., Rortveit, G., Bø, K., & Hunskaar, S. (2007). Urinary incontinence during pregnancy. *Obstetrics & Gynecology*, 109(4), 922-928.

Childbirth can also damage the pelvic muscles and tissues that are stretched during a vaginal delivery. The amount of damage depends upon the number of prior pregnancies, the type of delivery, the weight of the baby, the length of labor, and the length of time the mother had to push. If the pelvic muscles and tissues do not heal completely, the uterus and bladder neck may lose their support, and uterine prolapse may eventually result.

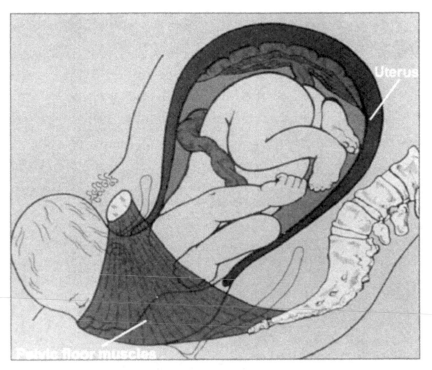

Diagram of Pelvic Floor Muscles Involved in Childbirth. Reprinted with permission. *The Urinary Incontinence Sourcebook.* McGraw Hill Education, Copyright 1999.

TECH TERMS

Uterine prolapse is when the uterus falls into the space occupied by the vagina.

As a baby descends the birth canal, the pudendal nerve may become damaged, leading to incontinence.

TECH TERMS

The **pudendal nerve** controls the muscles of the pelvic floor that surround the birth canal.

Bladder control problems may be caused by a delivery in which forceps are necessary.

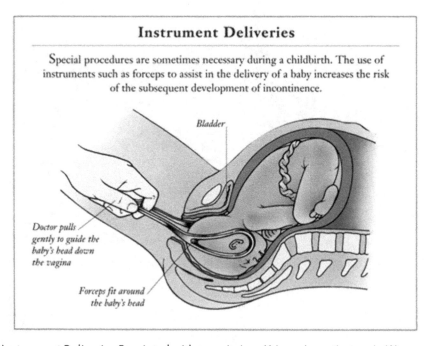

Instrument Deliveries

Special procedures are sometimes necessary during a childbirth. The use of instruments such as forceps to assist in the delivery of a baby increases the risk of the subsequent development of incontinence.

Bladder

Doctor pulls gently to guide the baby's head down the vagina

Forceps fit around the baby's head

Instrument Deliveries Reprinted with permission. *Urinary Incontinence in Women.* American College of Family Physicians, Home Medical Guides, p. 20, fig. "Instrument Deliveries." Copyright, 2000. Dorling Kindersley.

TECH TERMS

An **episiotomy** is an incision doctors sometimes make preceding childbirth to the perineum, the muscle between the vagina and rectum, to enlarge the vaginal opening, thus making it easier for the baby to emerge.

Problems with continence can also be caused by the episiotomy, the lying-down position in which women labor, and the necessity of pushing uphill during childbirth.

After childbirth, many women choose to breastfeed to pass on certain antibodies to their child, to provide better nutrition for their child, and to help burn off the weight gained during pregnancy. Breastfeeding, however, delays the normal functioning of the ovaries, delays the resumption of menstruation, and, therefore, causes estrogen levels to remain lower than normal. The estrogen-sensitive tissues in the pelvis will take longer to heal, and this may lead to incontinence.

Q&A

Is a caesarean section preferable to a vaginal delivery in order to prevent stress incontinence?

In all probability, the pressure of the contents of a pregnancy over the course of the nine-month gestation period is as responsible for pelvic nerve and muscle damage as the type of delivery. There is no doubt that pushing out a baby causes damage and that a woman with a personal or strong family history of pelvic floor relaxation may be counseled for an elective caesarean section. Pelvic nerve and muscle damage, however, may also occur with a caesarean section. It is important to note that caesarean section does not prevent incontinence.

Pelvic Surgery

Pelvic surgery can occasionally result in injury to pelvic muscles or nerves by overstretching them or by causing scar tissue that prevents them from functioning properly. Those who have undergone surgery (especially women who have had a hysterectomy) have a greater risk of subsequently suffering from incontinence.[32]

Menopause

As a woman enters menopause, the ovaries stop functioning, and estrogen levels fall dramatically. The estrogen-sensitive muscles of the pelvic floor (levator muscles) and tissues in the pelvis become thin, weaken, and atrophy (waste away). The bladder, bowels, and uterus lose their support due to a loss of collagen and eventually cause vaginal prolapse (dropping). Hormone replacement therapy may help reverse some of these bodily changes but cannot totally alleviate the problem. Once collagen has weakened, it can never regain its strength.

Low estrogen levels can result in vaginitis, a condition in which the vaginal walls become thin and the vagina becomes irritated and inflamed, causing soreness and itching. Bacterial levels within the vagina may also change. The resulting discomfort may lead to increased sensitivity around the urethra and to more frequent urination.

Topical vaginal estrogen is prescribed for patients with incontinence and vaginal atrophy (thinning of vaginal tissues). Vaginal estrogen can be prescribed in one of three different forms: cream, tablet, or ring. Vaginal estrogen has been associated with improved continence.[33] Oral estrogen may actually worsen incontinence and is, therefore, not prescribed.[34]

---

32 Mardon, RE, Halim, S, et al 2005. Management of Urinary Incontinence in Medicare Managed Care Beneficiaries. Journal of the American Medical Association. March 2005. 293(8):935–948.

33 Robinson, D., & Cardozo, L. D. (2003). The role of estrogens in female lower urinary tract dysfunction. *Urology*, 62(4), 45-51.

34 Hendrix, S. L., Cochrane, B. B., Nygaard, I. E., Handa, V. L., Barnabei, V. M., Iglesia, C., ... & McNeeley, S. G. (2005). Effects of estrogen with and without progestin on urinary incontinence. *Jama*, 293(8), 935-948.

TECH TERMS

Collagen is a protein in the skin that supports it. We always think about replacing the collagen in the skin on our faces, but collagen loss in the skin in other places also has a great impact.

Medications
Some prescription drugs and other over-the-counter drugs may cause incontinence during their use:

Drug	Example (Brand Name)
Diuretics (water pills)—may increase urine volume	Dyazide, Lasix, Esidrex, Maxide
Sedatives/muscle relaxants—may cause urgency, frequency, or decreased sensation to urinate	Valium, Librium, Ativan
Narcotics—may cause decreased sensation to urinate	Percocet, Demerol
Opiates—have narcotic effects	morphine
Antihistamines—may cause urinary retention/ weak stream	Benadryl
Antipsychotics/ antidepressants—may cause urinary retention	Haldol, Elavil, Prolixin, Prozac

Decongestants—may cause urinary retention/weak stream	Sudafed, Dexatrim, Entex
Anticholinergics (drugs used to stop bladder spasms)—may cause retention	Detrol, Ditropan, Sanctura
Cold remedies—may cause urinary retention/weak stream	Nyquil, Theraflu, Alka Seltzer Plus Cold Relief, Afrin long-lasting nose drops

Now, don't stop taking any of these drugs or flush them down the toilet if you need them. Before you do anything rash, consult your doctor, who will know how to proceed. Just be aware of the contraindications (situations in which the drug would not be prescribed, or when ingesting it would be harmful for you) for the above-mentioned medications if you are experiencing bladder problems or discomfort.

Low Fluid Intake

Wouldn't you bet me a package of adult diapers that limiting your intake of fluids would help reduce incontinence? Well, you'd be wrong, and I'd be going home with a product I no longer need. But you could argue that if you reduce the amount of beverages you consume daily that your kidneys would produce less urine. You'd be correct in that respect.

What you'd be overlooking, however, is that when you don't drink enough, your urine becomes highly concentrated. It turns a deep, dark yellow, smells a lot, and at that point becomes a bladder irritant. This can cause more frequent urination and bladder infections. Keeping your body properly hydrated will also help prevent constipation, another cause of incontinence. Fluid restriction as a means of curbing incontinence is considered only for patients with abnormally high fluid intake.[35]

---

35 Jackson SL, Weber AM, Hull TL, Mitchinson AR, Walters MD. 1997. Fecal incontinence in women with urinary incontinence and pelvic organ prolapse. Obstet Gynecol 89(3):423–7.

High Fluid Intake

Slow down! You don't want to go overboard with your intake of fluids. You don't need to walk around with a water bottle always in your hand. If you don't want to constantly run to the nearest restroom, limit your intake of alcohol, caffeinated coffee or tea, and sodas, because alcohol, caffeine, and carbonated beverages may serve as bladder irritants.

Q&A

How much fluid intake should I have on a daily basis?
You may have heard that you should have eight, eight-ounce glasses of liquid per day. When I went for physical therapy for my incontinence problems, the therapist explained to me that for my weight (124 pounds) that was the correct amount of fluid, but that number wouldn't work at all for my friend, who was 200 pounds. She suggested that a better rule of thumb (that takes weight into consideration) is to drink, in ounces per day, half of your body weight. That therapist cured me, and so I believe everything she says. Her words are gold. Trust me on that one.

Constipation

Think about the amount of pressure you put on your bladder when you strain and push to have a bowel movement. Preventing constipation by eating high-fiber foods and drinking plenty of water may help prevent incontinence. In a study of a group of women who experienced fecal incontinence, a positive association was seen between urinary incontinence and constipation.[36]

Smoking

Although the results of studies showing a relationship between nicotine and an overactive bladder are inconclusive, we all know that smoking is just not a

---

36   Handavl GH, Gold E, Robbins J. 2004. Progression and remission of pelvic organ prolapse—a longitudinal study of menopausal women. Am J Obstet Gynecol 190(1):27–32

healthy thing to do. Here are five potential side effects of smoking that may lead to incontinence:

1. Smokers cough, and they cough more frequently and more violently than non-smokers. Have you ever had a terrible cold and coughed so hard that you felt yourself leak? Violent coughing puts a tremendous amount of pressure on the pelvic muscle supports for the bladder, the urethra, and the vagina, thereby weakening them. Coughing can also cause urethral damage.

2. When a smoker inhales to fill his or her lungs, there is an increase in pressure within the abdomen, especially as the diaphragm lowers.

3. Nicotine can lead to increased bladder contractions, causing symptoms of urgency associated with an overactive bladder.

4. Smoking negatively impacts the already lowered estrogen levels of menopausal women by interfering with the proper functioning of the urethral sphincter. Bladder function is at increased risk because a smoker's collagen levels are decreased.

5. Smokers have an increased risk of developing bladder cancer.

Obesity

Obesity is definitely a risk factor for urinary incontinence because the additional pressure on the bladder by excess pounds can cause nerve and muscle damage. In one study, the prevalence of at least one weekly episode of stress incontinence increased by 10 percent for every five units of BMI (body mass index).[37] Weight reduction should be seriously considered for moderately or morbidly obese women with incontinence. In fact, urinary incontinence improves after weight loss surgery.[38]

---

37 Levy, R, Muller, N. Urinary Incontinence: Economic Burden and New Choices in Pharmaceutical Treatement. Advances in Therapy, Vol 23, No 4, July/August 2006.

38 Nygaard, C. C., Schreiner, L., Morsch, T. P., Saadi, R. P., Figueiredo, M. F., & Padoin, A. V. (2019). Urinary Incontinence and Surgery for Obesity and Weight-Related Diseases: Are There Predictors of Improvement?. *Obesity surgery*, 29(1), 109-113.

Q&A

How do I calculate my BMI?

BMI stands for "body mass index," a numerical value of your weight in relation to your height. The BMI number is a good indicator of healthy weights for adult men and women, regardless of body frame size. A BMI of 18.5 to 24.9 is generally considered healthy for most people. Research has indicated that lower BMIs (less than 18.5) and higher BMIs (25+) are associated with increased health risks. In general, obesity is defined as a BMI over 30, and morbid obesity as over 35.

Use the table below to find your BMI. Find your height in the left-hand column. Then look across the row to find your weight. Look at the top of the column to find your BMI (a number between 19 and 35). Note that pounds have been rounded off.

BODY MASS INDEX CHART

Height (inches)	19	20	21	22	23	24	25	26	27	28	29	30	31	32	33	34	35
58	91	96	100	105	110	115	119	124	129	134	138	143	148	153	158	162	167
59	94	99	104	109	114	119	124	128	133	138	143	148	153	158	163	168	173
60	97	102	107	112	118	123	128	133	138	143	148	153	158	163	168	174	179
61	100	106	111	116	122	127	132	137	143	148	153	158	164	169	174	180	185
62	104	109	115	120	126	131	136	142	147	153	158	164	169	175	180	186	191
63	107	113	118	124	130	135	141	146	152	158	163	169	175	180	186	191	197
64	110	116	122	128	134	140	145	151	157	163	169	174	180	186	192	197	204
65	114	120	126	132	138	144	150	156	162	168	174	180	186	192	198	204	210
66	118	124	130	136	142	148	155	161	167	173	179	186	192	198	204	210	216
67	121	127	134	140	146	153	159	166	172	178	185	191	198	204	211	217	223
68	125	131	138	144	151	158	164	171	177	184	190	197	203	210	216	223	230
69	128	135	142	149	155	162	169	176	182	189	196	203	209	216	223	230	236
70	132	139	146	153	160	167	174	181	188	195	202	209	216	222	229	236	243
71	136	143	150	157	165	172	179	186	193	200	208	215	222	229	236	243	250
72	140	147	154	162	169	177	184	191	199	206	213	221	228	235	242	250	258
73	144	151	159	166	174	182	189	197	204	212	219	227	235	242	250	257	265
74	148	155	163	171	179	186	194	202	210	218	225	233	241	249	256	264	272
75	152	160	168	176	184	192	200	208	216	224	232	240	248	256	264	272	279
76	156	164	172	180	189	197	205	213	221	230	238	246	254	263	271	279	287

Body Weight (pounds)

Caffeine

Caffeine, in general, is a diuretic as well as a bladder irritant for some people. Drinking or eating too many caffeinated products, including coffee and tea, carbonated soft drinks, sparkling water, and, alas, dark or milk chocolate, can also contribute to incontinence. Studies indicate that individuals who consume more than 204 mg of caffeine per day have increased urinary incontinence.[39] Patients can use a voiding diary to monitor their consumption of caffeinated products and fluids and make necessary adjustments to their diet.[40]

DOS AND DON'TS

When reducing your intake of caffeine, do proceed slowly over a period of several weeks. Trying to go cold turkey may result in withdrawal symptoms, such as strong or migraine headaches.

Caffeine is a known bladder irritant. It also acts as a diuretic, thereby stimulating the kidneys to produce more urine. Beware of the more than 1,000 over-the-counter drugs that contain caffeine, such as some pain medications intended to relieve symptoms of migraine headaches and menstrual cramps, as well as some substances to prevent sleepiness. Read labels before making a purchase.

Food Products

According to the National Association for Continence (NAFC), certain foods and non-caffeinated drinks are thought to contribute to the loss of bladder control. Although their effect on the bladder is not always understood, eliminating one or all of the items may help prevent bladder leakage. These products include the following foods and beverages:

39   Rohner TJ, Rohner JF. 1997. Urinary Incontinence in America: The social significance. In P. D. O'Donnel (ed.), Urinary Incontinence. St. Louis (MO): Mosby Yearbook, Inc.
40   Gleason, J. L., Richter, H. E., Redden, D. T., Goode, P. S., Burgio, K. L., & Markland, A. D. (2013). Caffeine and urinary incontinence in US women. *International urogynecology journal*, 24(2), 295-302.

- Acidic fruits: apples and apple juice, cantaloupe, citrus fruits and juices, grapes, guavas, peaches, pineapples, plums, and strawberries
- Alcoholic beverages, including wine and beer
- Any product containing an artificial sweetener
- Carbonated beverages that do not contain caffeine
- Coffee or tea (decaffeinated)
- Corn syrup
- Honey
- Milk and milk products
- Spicy foods, sugar, tomatoes and tomato-based products, vinegar
- Vitamins: B Complex and C (ascorbic acid)

BELIEVE IT OR NOT

I have been training with Jimmy, my personal "physical taskmaster," at the neighborhood gym for about seven years. Jimmy is not your run-of-the-mill trainer. He doesn't expect results; he demands them. He is merciless. If you don't achieve your goals (weight control, strength, body symmetry) in a timely fashion, you get a backroom lecture you don't want to hear. After a session with Jimmy, I am totally and completely wiped out for the rest of the day.

One day I decided that I would try to beat the intense fatigue I was experiencing by purchasing one of those new, flavored, vitamin-enriched power waters promising to give you all the energy you need. I tried the raspberry. I tried the lemon. I tried the orange. The taste was great, but the drinks did nothing to quench my thirst, improve my gym performance, or combat my exhaustion. I did notice, however, that about an hour after having a bottle of one of those waters, I had to make far too many trips to the bathroom to urinate. I never researched what the drinks contained, but I gave them up in favor of just plain tap water. Miraculously, that's all it took to regain control of my bladder.

High-Impact Physical Activities

Are you a female jock? Heed my words! High-impact physical activities, whether recreational or occupational, can cause increased pressure on the bladder because of the shaking movements and increased pull on the urinary organs. It is believed that approximately one-third of women who participate in these activities are subject to some degree of stress incontinence. Weak urethral muscles allow small amounts of urine to leak out. Sports that may increase pressure on the bladder include: running, jogging, jumping, power walking, high-impact aerobics, gymnastics, tennis, basketball, volleyball, handball, horseback riding, bodybuilding with heavy weights, karate, judo, and lifting heavy objects. Low-risk sports and activities include: swimming, yoga, low-impact aerobics, and bicycling.

DOS AND DON'TS

Do start doing Kegels at an early age. Even teenagers participating in high-impact physical activities can experience leakage.

Urinary Tract/Bladder Infection

Unfortunately for us gals, our anatomy is our destiny. Because our urethra is so short (three to five centimeters), it is very easy for bacteria to travel the small distance from our anus to our urethra and enter our bladder, especially if we aren't careful about wiping from front to rear. Bacteria may also be pushed into our bladder during sexual intercourse. An overgrowth of bacteria in the urine is an indication of a urinary tract infection (UTI), a.k.a. cystitis, a.k.a. bladder infection. Women at risk for a UTI may: void infrequently, allowing for a buildup of bacteria in their stagnant urine that can inflame the bladder or infect the urethra; be lax about wiping properly after a bowel movement; use a diaphragm that irritates them or that is improperly cleaned; and/or engage in rough sex that bruises the urethra or causes swelling and inflammation in the vaginal area.

DOS AND DON'TS

Do keep your prescribed antibiotic on hand if you are prone to frequent urinary tract infections. It's far better to be safe than sorry.

You will know when you have a UTI, because you will feel the urge to urinate very frequently, yet you will generally void only small amounts of urine. You may also experience burning, pain, or dysuria. A UTI is diagnosed by means of urinalysis, which detects the presence of bacteria in the urine. The infection is then treated with an antibiotic. Once you've had a UTI, you will never forget the uncomfortable, unpleasant experience.

TECH TERMS

Dysuria is pain or difficulty in urinating commonly caused by inflammation or infection.

Here are some tips that will help prevent a UTI:

- Drink lots of liquid to flush bacteria out of your body.
- Wear cotton underwear—it breathes and, therefore, doesn't provide a good breeding ground for bacteria.
- Avoid tight clothing, which tends to make you sweat and promotes the growth of bacteria.
- Make sure you void frequently enough so that bacteria can leave your system.
- Wipe from front to rear.
- Avoid detergent bath additives and colored and perfumed soaps and toilet tissue: the dyes and perfumes may be irritating.
- Schedule frequent bathroom breaks. Don't try to "hold it in."

Q&A

How can I prevent getting a UTI after intercourse?

Emptying the bladder soon after intercourse helps to wash away any bacteria that may be lurking in the vaginal area. Also, since urinary infections can occur as the result of using a diaphragm and spermicide, and since many women are allergic to the most common spermicide, nonoxynol-9, an alternative contraceptive method may eliminate bladder problems.

BELIEVE IT OR NOT

I love my mom. She's a great lady. But I must admit that oh so many years ago, when I was just a little girl, she neglected to teach me the fine art of and proper technique for wiping myself after a bowel movement. Did anyone ever caution you to wipe only from front to rear to prevent dire consequences? I wish someone—anyone—had taken me aside and taught me.

In any event, I guess I just successfully winged it until that sultry summer eve when I was eighteen. I remember that night forty years ago as if it had occurred yesterday. My future husband and I were at my best friend, Cheryl's, house for our nightly game of Scrabble. I must humbly state that I generally trounced each of them by at least fifty points, and they were out to get me that night, in usual fashion.

We had hardly begun to play when I was overcome by an immediate need to urinate. That accomplished, I returned. I sat down, feigned playing with my tiles, and scored thirty-seven points. No sooner had I picked new letters when I had to void once more. So, off I trotted again. And again. And again. My panties must have been up and down a minimum of seventy-five times. This urge to urinate plagued me throughout the entire evening and completely destroyed my ability to focus on anything other than Cheryl's pink porcelain toilet. In the meantime, both of my adversaries, whose concentration was keen and faultless, managed to outscore me unmercifully.

I couldn't wait to get home and I spent the entire night awake on the bathroom bowl. The doctor's diagnosis was a UTI. I took the magic pills that make you pee an unsightly orange and stain your pristine new white cotton panties forever as a reminder of your unfortunate transgression. Needless to say, to avoid future infections, I have always wiped from front to rear and have remained infection-free.

Interstitial Cystitis

Interstitial cystitis is similar to a UTI (cystitis) in that it causes frequent urination and pain. Unlike a UTI, however, it is not caused by a bacterial infection, and its cause is, to date, unknown. Interstitial cystitis is a condition that affects mostly women and is typified by chronic inflammation, thickening, and scarring of the bladder lining that causes frequency and urgency and can cause the bladder lining to bleed into the urine. It can also change the bladder's capacity for the worse and increase bladder sensitivity.

TECH TERMS

A **cystoscopy** is a procedure used to diagnose urinary tract disorders, wherein a flexible microscope is inserted first into the urethra and then into the bladder, allowing for a direct view of both.

To diagnose interstitial cystitis, a cystoscopy is performed by a urologist, who administers anesthesia and examines the bladder wall by inserting a cystoscope (a small microscope) into the bladder. After the doctor has had a good look around, with the cystoscope still in place, the bladder is filled to capacity with water.

If interstitial cystitis is present, some bleeding will be observed in the bladder wall. The diagnosis can be confirmed by performing a biopsy of the bladder wall and examining it under a regular microscope. Currently there is no permanent treatment for interstitial cystitis, and treatments that offer relief vary in their success rates.

Illnesses and Medical Events

Certain diseases and medical events can cause the bladder to malfunction, resulting in incontinence:

Illness or Medical Event	Result
Alzheimer's	Deterioration of the muscular function of the bladder.
Bladder Cancer	Frequency and urgency due to irritation.
Bladder Fistula	Formation of a hole in the wall separating the bladder from the vagina. Allows urine to leak from the bladder directly into the vagina without being stored. Often results from prior pelvic surgery.
Bladder Stones	Pressure on bladder causes frequency and urgency to urinate.
Brain or Spinal Tumors	Urgency and frequency.
Congestive Heart Failure	Increased urine production.
Dementia	Mental deterioration hampers awareness of the need to void and to get to a bathroom on time.
Diabetes	Frequency due to excessive thirst and drinking. Damage to the nerve supply to the bladder, resulting in detrusor instability (an unstable bladder) or difficulty in emptying the bladder.

Diverticula	Formation of pouches that hold excess urine and become inflamed in the walls of the urethra or bladder. Increased abdominal pressure and displacement of the bladder neck.
Fibroid Tumors	Increased abdominal pressure and displacement of the bladder neck.
Hypercalcemia	Production of large amounts of urine due to excessive amounts of calcium in the blood.
Lower Back Problems and Herniated Discs	Pinching of the nerves in the mid to lower back (thoracic, lumbar, and spinal regions).
Multiple Sclerosis	Loss of muscle coordination, control, and strength that fluctuates.
Parkinson's Disease	Weakness of sphincter muscles. Rigidity of muscles hampers ability to get to a bathroom on time.
Pelvic Organ Prolapse	Damage to the support ligaments in the pelvis causes the bladder, the uterus, or the bowel to sag.
Rheumatoid Arthritis	Stiffness in joints hampers ability to get to a bathroom on time.
Spinal Cord Injury	Lack of sensory awareness of the need to void hampers ability to get to a bathroom on time.
Stroke	Lack of sensory awareness of the need to void hampers ability to get to a bathroom on time.

Anatomic and Neurologic Abnormalities

Certain anatomical and neurological abnormalities also place people at risk for incontinence.

An ectopic ureter (the tube that connects the bladder to the kidney) is one that is not in its correct place. It may not connect to the bladder and enters the urethra or the vagina instead. Because the bladder is bypassed, leakage will occur.

Spina bifida is a birth defect in which the individual does not feel the urge to urinate when the bladder contracts. The bladder will void unpredictably when full or when exposed to other stimuli, such as cold.

Mind Over Matter, Mind Over Bladder

Although many of us tend to pooh-pooh them, emotional problems such as anxiety, confusion, depression, nervousness, or stress can lead to or aggravate already existing bladder problems and incontinence. As far-fetched as it may sound, it is essential to keep a clear, sound mind to maintain good bladder function. Anxiety, confusion, depression, nervousness, or stress can change your bladder habits and make you unaware of your bladder needs. Messages between your nervous system, your urinary tract muscles, and your brain must coordinate properly if you are to stay continent. So one of the keys to staying dry is to maintain good mental health.

Time To Go

How do you know when it is time to see your doctor? The National Association for Continence lists the ten warning signs of bladder problems. If you see your symptoms on this list, it's time to make an appointment with your physician:

1. Leakage of urine that prevents activities.
2. Leakage of urine that causes embarrassment.
3. Leakage of urine that began or continued after an operation, hysterectomy, or caesarean section.
4. Inability to urinate.
5. Urinating more frequently than usual without a proven bladder infection.
6. Need to rush to the bathroom and/or the loss of urine if you do not "arrive in time."
7. Pain related to filling the bladder and/or pain related to urination (in the absence of a bladder infection).
8. Frequent bladder infections.
9. Progressive weakness of the urinary stream with or without a feeling of incomplete bladder emptying.

10. Abnormal urination or changes in urination related to a nervous system abnormality (stroke, spinal cord injury, MS, etc.).

The Wrap-Up

- Physical conditions affect urinary frequency and urgency.
- Risk factors for bladder-control problems and incontinence include: gender and age, diet and exercise, lifestyle choices, illnesses and medical events, and anatomical and neurological abnormalities.
- Good mental well-being is essential to bladder control and continence.

4

Checking the Plumbing

Chapter Highlights

- Self Help
- Selecting a Doctor
- Basic Exams
- More Extensive Urodynamic Tests (a.k.a. urodynamics)
- The Wrap-Up

From early on, I knew that my plumbing was faulty, at best. I tried everything from stuffing toilet paper into my undies to purchasing extra-absorbent pads in an attempt to conceal the constant flow between and down my legs. Nothing came even remotely close to being effective. No matter what product I used, I overflowed. The problem was humiliating and not one to be discussed with one's mother, sister, or best girlfriend. I mean, really. How do you tell someone who thinks you're great that you constantly pee in your panties? So, I suffered in silence for an inordinately long amount of time.

But you don't have to do that. You don't have to hide your problem as I did. I'm here to help you and to show you that there are wonderful, compassionate medical professionals out there who can make your problem go away rather quickly.

Self Help

It's the twenty-first century and still only one out of four women with incontinence seeks medical help! And not only that, but medical studies show that the average time between the development of symptoms and the time a woman sees her doctor is seven years![41] You have got to help change that depressing statistic now.

Too many women believe that incontinence is a normal consequence of aging and/or that it is not treatable. They fail to understand that many causes of incontinence are reversible. More than 50 percent of women who suffer are too ashamed and embarrassed to consult medical professionals, who are an ideal source of information, education, treatment options, and support. Instead, these women alter their lifestyles to minimize leakage: they turn automatically to absorbent products without realizing that treatment is readily available to them; they avoid certain activities; they plan their daily excursions around the restrooms that will be available to them; and, in general, they become socially isolated. The personal cost of incontinence is reflected in a diminished quality of life and an increase in depression. Incontinence adversely affects physical functions (e.g., walking, lifting, engaging in sports, sex), daily activities (e.g., work, household chores), social interactions (e.g., visiting family and friends), productivity at work, personal hygiene, and a woman's emotional well-being. It's obvious, now more than ever, that it is time for incontinence to come out of the water closet for good![42]

Now, before you don your hat and coat and trot on over to your primary healthcare physician's office, consider the following list of things you can try to help yourself:

- Don't rush to get off the potty! Take your time. Void, take a rest, stand up, and then try again to make sure that you've completely emptied your bladder. You may even try to push on your bladder with your fingers to make sure you've gotten as much out as possible.
- I can't say this enough: wipe from front to back to avoid a urinary tract infection.
- Skip the sexy bubble bath, which might allow germs to travel from your anus to your bladder and cause an infection. Take showers instead.

41   Rabin JM, Stern JR. 2002. In You're Never Too Old to Have Fun—Tips on Staying Young and Being Healthy. New York:Stern/Greco Publishers. p 17.
42   Diokno A, Brock B, Brown M, Herzog A. 1986. Prevalence of urinary incontinence and other urological symptoms in the noninstitutionalized elderly. J Urol 136:1022–5.

- Drink enough fluids per day: half your weight in ounces of water should do the trick. Cut down drastically on caffeine, alcohol, and diet beverages that contain artificial sweeteners.
- Avoid foods and medications containing caffeine.
- Avoid medications that aggravate the bladder.
- Maintain a healthy weight.
- Exercise regularly.
- Do your Kegels! If these are unfamiliar to you, please read chapter 10.

If you've tried all these things and are still miserable, it's time to pay a visit to your family doctor so that your symptoms can be evaluated and treated.

Selecting a Doctor

If your primary care physician is on the ball, he or she should screen you for incontinence when you go for your annual physical. You shouldn't be embarrassed if your doctor asks you the following questions:

- Do you have issues with bladder control?
- Do you have trouble holding your urine?
- Do you feel that you empty completely?
- How often do you urinate during the day?
- How often do you wake at night to urinate?
- How much fluid do you drink per day?
- Are you constipated?
- Have you accidentally leaked urine with a physical activity such as coughing, sneezing, lifting, or exercising?
- How large an amount of urine do you lose?
- Have you felt a sudden urge to urinate that did not allow you to get to the toilet fast enough?
- Do you have pain or burning when you urinate?
- Does your bladder feel empty after you urinate?
- Do you feel any dropping of your bladder or uterus, and do you feel any bulging from your vagina?

- Do you feel pulling or pressure in your pelvis, especially when you've remained standing for a long period of time?
- Do you wear protective pads even though you don't want to?
- Have your sexual habits changed?

Before assuming that incontinence is actually the culprit, make sure that your doctor checks to see if you are suffering from a bladder or urinary tract infection (UTI) because these may give you similar symptoms. If you are experiencing urgency and/or frequent urination, pain in the area above your pubic bone or in your back, and/or fever, see your physician sooner rather than later, because those are signs of a UTI.

To really discover whether your doctor is paying attention and is willing to listen, ask any questions you have about incontinence or your specific symptoms. Prepare for your visit by making a list of your questions in advance, not just about incontinence but about your other health issues as well. You'd be surprised how much you forget to say once the doctor is in the consultation room with you. Have you ever gotten out of the office and said to yourself: "Gee, I forgot to ask the doctor about my (fill in the blank)"? Of course you have. We all have! You might write out your questions ahead of time so you and your doctor can review them together.

In any case, you deserve a doctor who will spend time investigating your concerns, diagnosing your condition, helping you develop reasonable treatment goals, suggesting appropriate treatments, monitoring you, and providing encouragement. Most importantly, you deserve a doctor who is willing to refer you to a specialist when appropriate.

If your family doctor dismisses your problem, says it's a normal consequence of aging, insists that it's something you'll just have to learn to live with, or doesn't pursue the problem further, run—don't walk—out of the office and find a specialist who will listen to you.

DOS AND DON'TS

If you need a referral for an incontinence specialist, do contact the National Association for Continence (NAFC) in Charleston, South Carolina at (800) 252-3337 or online at www.nafc. org, where you can find a continence care specialist within a specified distance of your zip code. They will gladly refer you to a reputable doctor in your area, free of charge, if you call 1-800-BLADDER (252-3337). For a nominal fee, you can receive the excellent, informative NAFC publication "Quality Care," which addresses important concerns for those who experience incontinence.

You may also contact the American Urogynecologic Society (AUGS), located in Silver Spring, Maryland, which will be happy to provide you with a list of urogynecologists in your area. Call AUGS at (301) 273-0570 or go online to www.augs.org.

Other agencies that can help you find a continence provider are:

- ACOG (The American College of Obstetricians and Gy-necologists): (800) 673-8444, (202) 638-5577, or online at www.acog.org
- AUA (The American Urologic Association): (410) 689-3700 or online at www.AUAnet.org
- APTA (American Physical Therapy Association): (800) 999-2782
- Simon Foundation: (800) 237-4666, or online at www.si-monfoundation.org

The first step toward getting better is seeing a specialist who is knowledgeable about incontinence and can evaluate the type of incontinence from which you suffer.

What kind of medical professional can help you with your incontinence? The first person to consult is your primary care physician, who will diagnose and treat or rule out infection. If your physician isn't well-versed in the dynamics of incontinence, you may also seek help from your gynecologist, who can determine if you have problems in your pelvic area but will likely have had little training in urology. Or you can see a urologist, who will recognize and take care of bladder and urinary tract problems, but may not have had much training with respect to the female reproductive system. Geriatricians, some physical therapists, and nurse specialists also deal with bladder problems. Perhaps the best person to see, however, is a urogynecologist.

What type of physician is that? A urogynecologist is a doctor who specializes in evaluating and treating, both surgically and non-surgically, the urologic and gynecologic problems that women experience. Their expertise lies in their ability to effectively help women with the various conditions that cause pelvic organ and pelvic floor dysfunction.

TECH TERMS

Urologists are doctors with specialized training regarding the urinary tract. **Urogynecologists** are doctors with specialized training in both female urologic and gynecologic problems. They examine and treat conditions that affect the muscles and tissues that support female pelvic organs.

BELIEVE IT OR NOT

I secretly met with a male urologist for my bladder control problems when I was a young married woman, after I had just given birth to my first son. The doctor decided that he could cure me by stretching my urethra on three separate occasions. Foolishly, I believed him. I went the first time and looked on with trepidation as he stood poised with the needle of Novocain and the instrument he was going to insert. I didn't feel pain then, but boy was I in agony afterwards. It hurt and burned so much when I urinated that I screamed out loud and had to hold myself to try to prevent the searing pain. And the blue urine resulting from the antibiotic ruined several pairs of my finest sexy lace panties. Naïve woman that I was, I went back for the second round of stretching. Although I was told that it would get better each time, it was just as bad. No, I wasn't dumb enough to go back for the third time. I threw up my arms in despair and resigned myself to a lifetime of adult diapers.

Several years went by, and I again secretly decided to try another male urologist whom everyone raved about. He did all kinds of tests and concluded that if I didn't drink any fluids after 7:00 p.m., I'd be cured. That diagnosis cost me several hundred dollars but didn't help my incontinence one bit. Once again, I gave up.

More and more years went by. Finally, my masseuse recommended a very highly regarded female urogynecologist. This doctor ran more tests than I want to remember. She didn't hurt me or give me silly advice. She talked to me. She examined me. She explained her diagnosis and then sent me for further treatment to a female physical therapist trained in urogynecology. It was a match made in heaven. Today, I am cured. You can be, too.

So how do you go about choosing the doctor who's right for you? The late humorist, columnist, and author Erma Bombeck once said, "Never go to a doctor whose office plants have died." Think about it: if the physician doesn't care enough to maintain the living things in her office, and if she can't keep those things alive, how much confidence can you have in this person?

I have always found that the best way to select a really good doctor is to get a referral from a friend or family member who has had a related problem and whose opinions I respect. But don't stop there. We're talking about your health and your comfort! Investigate thoroughly. Do you really want to see someone who graduated from the University of "Who Knows Where"? Find out about the doctor's credentials. You can look the doctor up in your state medical society's directory, which can be found in your public library; at your state medical society office; or simply by going online. Make sure that the physician is board certified and that his or her certification is current. Ascertain how much experience the doctor has and where he or she received it.

Find out with which hospitals your doctor is affiliated. Do you really want someone who practices at an unknown facility or at one of poor repute? Then do some research on the quality of care afforded by that facility. Also ask if the practitioner you would like to use accepts your medical insurance. If so, great! If not, only you can determine whether you want to look elsewhere or pay the out-of-pocket expenses.

The National Association for Continence (NAFC) provides the following list of questions (reprinted with permission) you should ask to ascertain the expertise of any urology specialist you plan on using:

1. Does the specialist have interest and training in the diagnosis and management of incontinence?
2. How long has he/she been focusing on the field of incontinence?
3. What sorts of medical problems have his/her incontinent patients had?
4. Does the specialist have the ability to do office testing of bladder function to help determine the cause of incontinence?
5. Do other health professionals refer incontinent patients to this specialist for treatment?
6. Does the specialist have experience in the treatment of patients who have had previous unsuccessful attempts at correcting their incontinence?
7. Is the specialist experienced with non-surgical forms of treatment for incontinence, such as pelvic muscle exercises, behavioral therapy, clean intermittent self-catheterization, etc.?
8. Can the specialist provide prescriptions for medication?
9. Does the specialist teach other health professionals about the diagnosis and treatment of incontinence?
10. Is the specialist experienced in the evaluation of patients for the implantation of devices such as the artificial urinary sphincter?
11. Is the specialist experienced in the evaluation and treatment of incontinence related to birth defects, diseases, and accidents that cause spinal injury or bladder damage?

12. If the incontinence cannot be cured, can the specialist or someone in the office tell you about printed information, support groups, and/or management alternatives that will make life with this condition more comfortable?

13. Does the specialist know about the Agency for Healthcare Policy and Research Guidelines for the Treatment of Urinary Incontinence in Adults and about the National Association for Continence?

14. Does the specialist have knowledge of local community resources, such as home delivery services?

I found the best doctor through a referral, and she took my insurance. This was the bargain of the century! She referred me to a pricey, yet extremely professional and competent physical therapist who wasn't on my plan. She was, however, worth her weight in gold. The four visits I needed cost less than 1,000 dollars. That was probably the best money I have ever spent.

BELIEVE IT OR NOT

I was plagued with incontinence for most of my life and never dreamed there was any recourse other than panty liners or diapers until one day …

Can you picture this? There I lie, naked as a jaybird, getting a full body massage from my seventy-five-year-old masseuse, Barbara, who had spent decades studying philosophy and transcendental meditation with an honest-to-goodness maharishi. Ambient sitar music quietly played in the background as we engaged in idle girlie chitchat. I was so comfortable and so relaxed until all of a sudden I felt it—you know—that immediate urge to jump off the table and make a beeline for the bathroom. I whipped off the sheets and left the warm, comfortable massage bed for the icy chill of a stark, tiled bathroom. Fortunately, I made it just in the nick of time.

When I had resettled myself, Barbara very gently alluded to my problem and, I couldn't help it, I told her the whole sad tale. She explained that her daughter had had a similar problem and, with the help of an excellent doctor, was now cured. Of course I took down the number, called from my cell the minute I could, and made the most important medical appointment of my life.

Basic Exams

Your doctor will first ask you about your symptoms, medical and surgical history, and family history, so make sure you've done your homework and kept a list of all your symptoms and problems. You will be questioned about your degree of discomfort, recent illnesses, and use of medications. Sometimes a simple change in prescription can cure incontinence.

Next comes the examination—not a fun experience. Your doctor will perform abdominal, pelvic, rectal, and neurological examinations. While some of the following tests may seem strange or uncomfortable, taking them is an early—and brief—step toward solving your incontinence:

- A urinalysis and a urine culture to check for infection, inflammation, crystals, or blood and/or sugar in the urine.
- A uroflowmetry test is used to measure postvoid residual urine volume (PVR). Done by catheter or bladder scan, this test determines how much urine is left in the bladder after voiding.
- A Q-Tip or cotton swab test determines the mobility of your urethra in relation to your bladder. This may or may not be a factor for incontinence or prolapse in your particular situation.
- A pad test determines the amount of leakage.
- A stress test checks for the loss of urine by determining how much, if any, leakage there is with walking, coughing, laughing, or bearing down.
- Bedside urodynamics obtains diagnostic information about the type of urinary incontinence without using electronic equipment.

- The Valsalva leak point pressure (VLPP) measures the competency of the urethra. (This test may be a part of the bedside urodynamics or the more complex "multichannel urodynamics" mentioned below).
- A multichannel urodynamics (UDS) or cystometrogram (CMG) is a testing procedure that measures the capacity, irritability, elasticity, and leakage of the bladder. UDS measures the pressure and volume of the bladder as it fills as well as the rate of flow as it empties.
- An intravenous urogram examines the anatomy of the kidneys, ureters, and bladder.
- Cystoscopy or cysto-urethroscopy enables the doctor to see the inside of the urethra and the inside wall of the bladder. A cystoscope is a long, narrow tube with a light and camera lens.
- An electromyogram (EMG) evaluates whether the pelvic muscles are contracting and relaxing properly. The test measures this by checking the connection between the nerves that send messages (electrical signals) to the muscles.

DOS AND DON'TS

Don't allow incontinence to affect you and your family or your health and quality of life. Take action now! An open dialogue with your doctor is important during the evaluation and treatment processes.

In order to properly diagnose the cause and extent of your incontinence, a specialist will have to check your abdomen, your pelvis, your rectum, and your nervous system. By examining your abdomen, the physician can tell if any masses are present (and causing pressure), if your bladder is full or tender (and not emptying properly), and if your bowel is not overly filled with stool (indicating that you are not constipated). A pelvic exam in both the standing and lying-down position will indicate that your internal organs are healthy and in their proper positions, that no prolapse (a downward dropping of the pelvic organs) has occurred, and that no masses are present. The strength of your pelvic floor muscles can also be determined. A rectal exam identifies any problems with constipation and fecal continence. Neurological testing will check your reflexes and will make sure that the nerves controlling your bladder, urethra, and pelvic floor are working properly.

DOS AND DON'TS

When you make an appointment to see a specialist, do make sure you bring along a list of all the medications (prescription and over-the-counter) and vitamin and herbal supplements you take. In advance of your visit to the specialist, keep another log (for at least twenty-four and up to forty-eight hours) listing your hourly fluid intake, the number of times you voided, the times at which you voided, any voiding or leakage events and the time at which they occurred, and the approximate amount voided. Show both of these records to the doctor.

Once these preliminary tests have been done, a **urinalysis** and urine culture will be performed to ascertain that your bladder problems aren't the result of an infection. In order to get an uncontaminated specimen, your specialist may ask you to provide a "midstream" sample. Here's what you'll have to do:

- Spread your labia (the lips of your vagina) with your fingers.
- Use the moist towelette that is provided and carefully wipe from front to back.
- Start to urinate in the toilet.
- Once you've released urine for a second or two, don't stop, and place the cup underneath you to catch the midstream flow.
- Remove the cup and finish voiding into the toilet.

White blood cells and/or bacteria in the urine generally indicate an infection, which can be treated with antibiotics. Hematuria or blood (red blood cells) in the urine may or may not be indicative of bladder cancer or bladder stones and will require further testing.

You may be asked to keep a voiding diary as mentioned above (anywhere from one to seven days) in which you note your fluid intake at specific times, the approximate amount of urine eliminated (through voiding or leakage), the times these events occurred, and your activity level at the time of the actual leakage. This is a simple way to show your specialist how your bladder is functioning and what tests should be considered next.

A **pad test** may be used to measure leakage and may be performed in the specialist's office or at home. Pad testing can be done over a period of time as short as twenty minutes or up to one hour: a sanitary napkin is weighed and then worn for twenty to sixty minutes, during which time the individual is asked to perform certain activities which may include:

- Walking briskly for three minutes.
- Sitting and then standing ten to twenty times.
- Walking up and down stairs for one to two minutes.
- Picking up objects from the floor five to ten times.
- Coughing twelve times (at various strengths; may be repeated).
- Running in place for one minute (may be repeated).

The pad is then removed and weighed again to calculate the amount of urine voided. A small loss may indicate stress incontinence, for example, while a greater loss may indicate unstable bladder contractions (detrusor instability), usually associated with the urge symptoms. Coloring agents may also be used to determine that the fluid lost is urine. This is called a dye test and is performed after a non-toxic dye is placed in the bladder. Any stain of dye on the pad following the test indicates that urine was lost during the test.

TECH TERMS

Detrusor instability refers to an unstable bladder, one in which the detrusor muscle (the muscle responsible for contracting the bladder so that urine can be voided) contracts involuntarily and for no apparent reason. This is associated with symptoms such as urge to void and urinary frequency (voiding more often than is considered the norm).

When the test is performed over a twenty-four hour period at home, pads are each worn for approximately two-hour intervals and then removed. Each is placed in a sealed bag, labeled separately with the date and time removed, and then returned to the doctor's office at the next visit.

A **Q-Tip** test can be performed in your doctor's office. While you are on the examining table, body reclined—with your legs up in those stirrups, of course—a Q-Tip lubricated with anesthetic gel is inserted into your urethra (the opening to your bladder). Don't worry. It doesn't hurt. You are then asked to cough and strain, and the doctor will observe how the cotton swab reacts. Too much movement of the Q-Tip may be indicative of a weak pelvic floor and weak urethral connective tissue, which may place a woman at risk for incontinence.

During your visit, your doctor may perform a **cough stress test.** You will be asked to come to the office with a full bladder and asked to cough in an upright and supine (lying-down) position. Then you may be asked to empty your bladder. This urine may be sent for various tests. You will also be asked to repeat this coughing maneuver with an empty bladder. If you lose urine with either a full or empty bladder, the diagnosis may be stress incontinence.

More Extensive Urodynamic Tests (a.k.a. urodynamics)

Urodynamic tests are performed by a urogynecologist or urologist to check the function of the bladder. They determine whether or not the relationship between pressure and volume in the bladder is normal as it fills and if the flow rate is normal as the bladder empties. It is a sophisticated way to reproduce bladder symptoms and to pinpoint specific problems.

TECH TERMS

Urodynamics or urodynamic testing (a.k.a. cystometrics) is a sophisticated way to reproduce bladder symptoms and to pinpoint specific problems in order to evaluate bladder function. It is the study of, and a series of tests determining how the bladder, urethra, and pelvic floor muscles function.

A **uroflowmetry** test may be the first test performed to ensure that you aren't abnormally retaining urine. Urine retention may be due to a problem with the nerves controlling the bladder and the pelvic floor or due to a bladder obstruction. A flowmeter measures the quantity of fluid voided per unit of time, which should be more than ten cc per second for women

TECH TERMS

The postvoid residual urine volume (PVR) is the amount of urine that remains in your bladder after you've voided. A PVR of more than 200 cc of urine indicates a problem.

Have you ever gone into the bathroom with a book that was thoroughly engrossing, sat down, gotten comfortable, voided completely (you thought), only to find that you were still not done urinating a half-hour later? And, of course, before finally getting up you void again—not a lot, a few drops or an ounce or two, just enough to make it worth the effort. It is unusual for the bladder to empty completely, and the postvoid residual urine volume (PVR), the amount of urine left in your bladder after you've urinated, can be measured by catheterization or ultrasound.

If urodynamics (UDS) or bladder testing is to be performed, within a few minutes after you've urinated, a catheter may be inserted into your bladder. This enables the doctor to drain and measure any remaining urine. This urine may be sent for testing to rule out infection or other problems. A reading of one to three ounces is normal (although it may be higher in older individuals). A **bedside urodynamics** test is performed without using any electronic equipment. A catheter is inserted into your bladder, which is then filled with fluid. The catheter is connected to a large, empty syringe, which is held upright. The bladder is then filled, two ounces at a time, with sterile saline or water. The syringe is carefully monitored. As the bladder is filling, the doctor will ask you to report what you feel. If you feel an overwhelming urge to urinate, and the doctor notices a sudden rise in the level of fluid in the syringe, you may be suffering from urge incontinence. When the bladder is full, the catheter is removed, and the doctor can then check again for prolapse. The doctor will instruct you (with a full bladder) to cough and to bear down in order to check for any signs of stress incontinence.

I have had a test known as a **multichannel urodynamics (UDS) or complete cystometry**, and I'm still not sure which is more embarrassing: peeing in my pants or peeing in a toilet where everyone is watching and measuring my output. Fortunately, the doctor and nurses who attended to me were extraordinarily compassionate and had a great sense of humor. That made all the difference in the world to me, and somehow I managed to chat and laugh my way through the experience.

UDS measures the relationship between pressure and volume when the bladder is filling and is used to determine whether or not this relationship is normal. At first, I had to urinate into a special toilet that measured my urinary flow rate (see uroflowmetry below). Then special detectors (very small catheters that measure pressure and are able to fill the organ with fluid as needed) were placed in my bladder and my rectum. I reported my symptoms as my bladder was filled slowly with sterile water through this catheter. That took about five minutes. During that time, the pressures from the detectors were recorded. Can you imagine that—with all these wires running out of me they made me cough and jump? You know, of course, that I leaked like crazy.

Finally, they let me urinate again while they measured my bladder pressure and recorded my flow rate (see uroflowmetry below). This is the best way, they told me, to figure out if I had stress, urge, or mixed (both types) incontinence.

In other words, I was finally going to have a diagnosis! **Cystometry** is used to determine whether incontinence is the result of involuntary bladder contractions (urge incontinence or detrusor instability), weak pelvic muscles or urethral sphincter (stress incontinence), or both (mixed incontinence) and whether there is pain or discomfort when the bladder fills or empties.

TECH TERMS

Cystometry is the measurement of the pressure and volume of the bladder both when full and when emptying. The **cystometer**, the machine that performs this urodynamic test, produces a graph called a **cystometrogram.**

Valsalva leak point pressure (VLPP) is a reliable test that is easy to perform. It measures the lowest abdominal pressure required during a stress activity (such as coughing) that would cause the urethra to open and, therefore, leak. To perform this test, catheters are placed in the bladder and rectum (see cystometry above). The bladder is filled with sterile water or saline to at least one-half its capacity. You'll be asked to slowly cough or bear down until leakage is seen and measured by the cystometer. Pressure within the abdomen is measured by means of a small rectal balloon. The smallest increase in pressure that results in leakage is called the VLPP. A normal urethra will not leak at any abdominal pressure. For purposes of reliability, this study is performed at least twice. If you leak during this test, you probably suffer from stress incontinence. Generally, both **UDS** and **video urodynamic tests (VUDS)** are performed if bedside cystometrics were inconclusive.

A video urodynamic test, or VUDS (cystometry used in conjunction with x-ray imaging to evaluate and examine the position of the bladder neck when leakage occurs during exertion), is very helpful for women who have undergone surgery or who have complicated problems. While it may be the most precise method for determining and classifying stress urinary incontinence, it requires x-ray equipment and facilities with lead-lined rooms. These are not always readily available.

TECH TERMS

Uroflowmetry tests for blockages in the urethra and abnormal voiding patterns and measures the strength, volume, and smoothness of urinary flow and the length of time it takes to urinate and to stop urinating.

I've also had a **uroflowmetry** test, which is a simple, non-invasive procedure that indicates how well the bladder and urethra work together and if there are any obstructions. For this test, the individual urinates on a uroflow chair (which is a commode equipped with a special meter). The urinary stream is evaluated according to its strength, volume, and smoothness. Also noted is how long it takes the individual to void and to stop voiding. This is not a physically difficult test: there is no pain. For me, it was a bit embarrassing, however, because the clinician was right there with me while I was relieving myself. (She did, however, offer to step out of the room.) I think it really helps to know that everyone involved in these testing procedures has done this many times and they've seen and heard everything. So while you are totally mortified, for them, this is just second nature and no big deal.

How Cystoscopy Works

A **cystoscopy** may also be performed to ensure that the inside of the urethra and bladder are healthy. The cystoscope is a long, narrow metal or flexible lit tube with a camera lens. Prior to insertion, anesthetic jelly is inserted into the urethra to make the exam virtually painless. The scope is then inserted into the urethra and into the bladder while the doctor examines these organs. During the test, water is used to distend the bladder so that the doctor can more easily visualize the inside of these organs. Any abnormalities of the bladder or urethra such as blockages, scar tissue, stones, irritation, or polyps are noted. This test is usually reserved for people who have had blood in their urine, repeated bladder infections, or urge incontinence that does not respond to treatment.

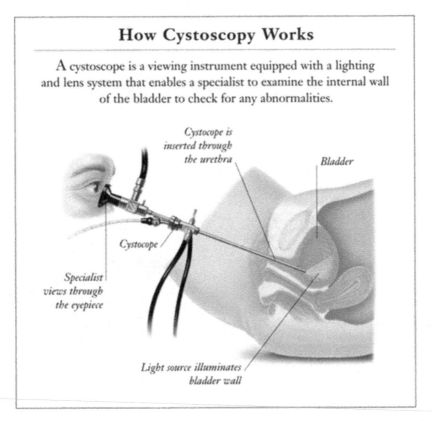

How Cystoscopy Works

A cystoscope is a viewing instrument equipped with a lighting and lens system that enables a specialist to examine the internal wall of the bladder to check for any abnormalities.

Cystocope is inserted through the urethra

Bladder

Cystocope

Specialist views through the eyepiece

Light source illuminates bladder wall

Reprinted with permission. *Urinary Incontinence in Women.* American College of Family Physicians, Copyright 2000, Dorling Kindersley.

The Wrap-Up

- If you think you have a problem with incontinence, first closely monitor your toileting habits and patterns.
- Take precautions to prevent bladder infections.
- Investigate and then select a competent, sympathetic doctor with good credentials who is affiliated with an outstanding hospital.
- If you need a referral, contact one of the organizations that specializes in problems with incontinence.

- Get a complete physical when you see your doctor.
- Initially, a voiding diary, a urinalysis, and a pad test may be used to determine the extent of your problem.
- Cystometrics, including a test for postvoid residual urine volume (PVR), uroflowmetry, and/or cystoscopy, will also be used to diagnose the nature of your problem.

5

Diagnosis: Stress Incontinence

Chapter Highlights

- Stresses and Pressures
- Symptoms
- Causes
- Treatment
- The Wrap-Up

Your cold has finally blossomed: your eyes are watery, your nose is running, and your ears are clogged. All of a sudden, quite without warning, from the depths of your insides you let out a loud, raspy, bronchial cough that seems to make the walls shake. Then you feel it. Oh my goodness, no! It's there! That one little drop that managed to escape is now spreading all over the bottom of your cotton panties and is threatening to penetrate your new camel suede pants. You feel another cough looming and realize you've got to do something—and fast! Adult women expect their bladders to behave all the time. They may not realize that activities such as coughing, sneezing, laughing, jumping, and heavy lifting, activities that put pressure on weakened bladder or pelvic muscles, can cause leakage. Remember, leakage can only occur when the pressure in the bladder exceeds the pressure in the urethra!

TECH TERMS

Stress incontinence refers to the involuntary loss of urine associated with activities that increase pressure in the abdomen, such as coughing, laughing, sneezing, or physical exertion.

Stresses and Pressures

Generally when we think about stress and pressure, we are referring to the emotions we feel as a result of life's daily trials and tribulations. Incontinence, however, is a very real reaction to physical stress and pressure on muscles and tissues in our body.

Stress incontinence is the most common type of incontinence, accounting for between 40 and 50 percent of all cases reported by women.[43] Considering that most cases are treatable, it is unfortunate that some women, out of fear, ignorance, shame, embarrassment, societal pressures, and guilt, may wait as long as seven years before seeking medical help![44]

The majority of people with stress incontinence are women. Why is this?

- Men don't have a uterus. They don't carry babies for nine months. They don't go through the trauma of delivery; they suffer no nerve or tissue damage, and their pelvic muscles do not get stressed and stretched.
- Men have longer urethras than women so, at least in theory, they have a longer "tube" that works with and closes against bladder pressure.
- Men don't go through menopause, which weakens pelvic floor and vaginal muscles and leads to stress incontinence.
- Men who do suffer from stress incontinence may have had prostate or another type of pelvic/bladder surgery that may have caused weakening or loss of the urethral sphincter's muscle function.

Technically speaking, there are two types of stress incontinence:

---

43   Op. cit. "What is Incontinence?"
44   Nygaard, et al. Is urinary incontinence a barrier to exercise in women? 2005. Obstet Gynecol 106(2):307.

- external sphincter insufficiency
- intrinsic sphincter deficiency

External sphincter insufficiency (ESD), the most common of the two types of stress incontinence, causes leakage when the abdominal muscles tighten and create abdominal pressure against the bladder and urethra (during coughing, laughing, sneezing). A well-supported urethra will not leak. For someone with stress incontinence, however, the pelvic floor muscles and the connective tissue that supports the bladder and urethra are so worn that when the stress of a cough occurs, bladder pressure (from the stress pressure in the abdomen) exceeds pressure in the urethra (pushed down and out of the abdominal compartment) and causes leakage.

Intrinsic sphincter deficiency (ISD) is a less common form of stress incontinence and may happen after pelvic surgery, an anti-incontinence procedure, a vaginal birth, or in conjunction with a neurological problem. Something malfunctions in the urethra and causes it to refuse to stay tightly closed. Do you know what a Chinese finger puzzle is? It's a woven tube of straw. You put a finger into each end of the tube, and if you pull simultaneously on your fingers, they get stuck. Just as with the puzzle, imagine that the urethra is closed shut by its sphincter, or closing muscle. The bladder may be well-anchored, the pelvic muscles and connective tissue may support all of the pelvic organs, and yet, when this muscle (sphincter) doesn't work, the urethra doesn't close properly. Leakage occurs as a result of this, because the pressure in the bladder is then greater than the pressure in the urethra.

Something as insignificant as a hiccup, or as taxing as aerobic exercise, can present a bladder challenge. Without warning, and in a flash, a person suffering from stress incontinence can be faced with an extremely embarrassing situation—the spot that spreads!

Stress incontinence is also referred to as:

1. genuine stress incontinence
2. external sphincter incompetence (ESD)
3. urethral insufficiency/intrinsic sphincter deficiency (ISD)

BELIEVE IT OR NOT

My girlfriends are like camels—they can hold in their urine all day! Me, I laugh and I pee. I sneeze and I pee. I cough and I pee. I run and I pee. Just about any unexpected, sudden pressure makes me lose control. Usually I escape with losing just a little trickle of urine—enough to remind me that I'll be a little damp for a while and that I shouldn't have worn my $50 white French lace panties that day.

Of course, if the pressure is great, like when I laugh out loud, then the floodgates open, and I have to bolt for the nearest bathroom. I cannot begin to count the number of times I have had to wring out my undies in a ladies room and then line them with wads of toilet paper because I didn't think I'd need a protective pad that day. I have ruined clothing, sofas, chairs, and car seats. Fortunately for me, I received excellent medical help and have learned to successfully deal with both problems. If I could do it, anyone can.

Having stress incontinence is like having occasional faulty plumbing. Your sphincter muscles (for ISD) and/or pelvic floor muscles (for ESD) are not working effectively and can't properly control a leak in your bladder. In some cases, this weakness can be so severe that standing or walking, in addition to the other activities mentioned in this chapter, can cause frequent trips to the bathroom or voiding accidents.

Do you have stress incontinence? Take this simple test:

1. Do you lose urine when you laugh?
2. Do you lose urine when you sneeze?
3. Do you lose urine when you cough?
4. Do you lose urine when you exercise?
5. Do you lose urine when you engage in any of these physical activities: running, high-impact aerobics, tennis, low-impact aerobics, walking,

golf, bicycling, racquetball, swimming, lifting weights, moving furniture, vacuuming, mowing the lawn?

6. Do you lose urine when you lift heavy objects?
7. Do you lose urine when you walk?
8. Do you lose urine when you stand?
9. Do you lose urine after having had a hysterectomy or other pelvic surgery?

Did you answer yes to any of the above questions? If so, it's time to get evaluated by a urogynecologist or urologist, because you can be helped.

Q&A

Is incontinence during exercise unusual?
Studies show that more and more women in our increasingly health-conscious society experience incontinence when exercising—more than one out of three of those who have experienced childbirth and one out of seven of those who are childless have noted leakage during exercise. Curiously, incontinence during exercise was less common than when women performed more routine daily activities such as vacuuming or lifting heavy objects.[45]

Symptoms

Stress incontinence produces leakage to a lesser or greater degree depending on the severity of the case and the activities performed.

Minimal stress incontinence occurs when a person experiences leakage while engaging in rather rigorous activity, such as aerobic exercise or high-impact sports. Severe or strong coughing, sneezing, or laughing will also cause

---

45 Olsen AL, Smith VJ, Bergstrom JO, Colling JC, Clark AL. 1997. Epidemiology of surgically managed pelvic organ prolapse and urinary incontinence. Obstet Gynecol 89:501–6.

a problem. Moderate stress incontinence occurs with less demanding activities, such as standing up or walking. Severe stress incontinence occurs with very little activity at all, such as turning over in bed. If this sounds like you, the ISD type of stress incontinence may be the culprit.

DOS AND DON'TS

If you suffer from stress incontinence:
Don't
1. spend a lot of money on expensive pads and/or protective undergarments.
2. think that crossing your legs will work.
3. try to hold back a cough, sneeze, or laugh.
4. limit your physical activity.

Do
1. make an appointment with a urogynecologist for an evaluation.
2. get a second opinion if you feel that this is necessary or if you feel uncomfortable with your first opinion.
3. consider your options.

Causes

Stress incontinence in women may be caused by weakened pelvic muscles or connective tissue (fascia) or weakened urethral sphincter muscles. There are several different explanations for how these muscles lose their original good tone and, consequently, cause bladder accidents.

Weakened pelvic muscles (those that support the bladder, bladder neck, and urethra) are the primary cause of stress incontinence in women.

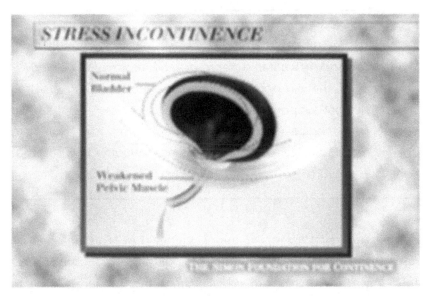

Reprinted with permission. The Simon Foundation for Continence.

TECH TERMS

Urethral hypermobility refers to too much movement of the urethra, causing it to drop below the pelvic floor muscles during certain activities. This may or may not cause leakage.

When the support provided by the pelvic muscles is relaxed or lost, the bladder neck and urethra may shift, sag, or drop into a lower position during periods of activity, thus causing pressure on the bladder neck area. The pressure on the bladder will exceed the pressure on/in the urethra. If the bladder neck or urethra opens briefly, leakage occurs.

Q&A

What percentage of women suffer from pelvic organ prolapse (POP)?
Studies show that 50 percent of women who have had children lose pelvic floor support resulting in prolapse. Of these, only 10–20 percent seek medical care for their symptoms. The true figures are unknown due to under-reporting and under-inquiring by both patients and doctors.[46]

Prolapse may cause the vagina, uterus, urethra, small intestine, and rectum to drop below their normal position, possibly causing stress incontinence. The prolapsed organs are covered with vaginal skin, so they just look like big bulges in any of the five areas mentioned above. If you have POP, you may feel as though you are "sitting on an egg." There are five main areas/types of prolapse, and you may have one or a combination of them:

- Cystocele—The bladder drops down into the vagina, resulting in incomplete emptying of the bladder and a possible urinary tract infection. A cystocele may become worse with time.
- Cystourethrocele—The lower part of the urethra drops down into the vagina. This is also usually associated with a cystocele.
- Uterine prolapse—The uterus and cervix drop down into the vagina, resulting in urinary urgency and frequency. If you have had a hysterectomy, your vagina may prolapse, because it is located in the middle compartment of your pelvic area above the (now removed) uterus.
- Enterocele—The small intestine drops into the vagina.
- Rectocele—The rectum protrudes into the vagina, resulting in incomplete rectal emptying.

---

46 American Urogynecologic Society (AUGS) Web site (www.augs.org), p 1–2.

The symptoms of prolapse include:
- lower back pain
- pelvic pressure and heaviness
- difficulty controlling urine and stool
- urinary urgency and frequency
- a dripping or bulging feeling in the vagina
- irritation of protruding tissue
- a feeling of "sitting on an egg"
- sexual dysfunction
- urinary retention

There are four different grades of prolapse, depending upon its severity:
- Grade 1: The sagging organ bulges toward the opening of the vagina.
- Grade 2: The sagging organ is halfway down the vaginal canal.
- Grade 3: The sagging organ is at the opening of the vagina.
- Grade 4: The sagging organ drops out of the vagina.

DOS AND DON'TS

To use your muscles properly:
- Tighten them during strenuous activity.
- Tighten them when lifting heavy objects.
- Tighten them when coughing, sneezing, or laughing.

The causes of relaxed, weakened, or lost pelvic or sphincter muscle support, which may result in leakage and/or pelvic organ prolapse (POP), are:
- Pregnancy: the weight of the fetus puts pressure on the pelvic floor, causing the tissues to stretch or sag.
- Difficult childbirth: tissues are stretched or torn.
- Obesity: excess weight in the abdomen puts pressure on the bladder.

- Chronic constipation: the urethra is blocked and prevents the bladder from being completely emptied or the constant pressure of bearing down strains and weakens the muscles and connective tissues.
- Abdominal and vaginal surgery: tissues and nerves may be damaged.
- Menopause: hormonal changes, notably the decrease in estrogen, causes the tissues of the urethra to become thin. The urethral opening enlarges and allows urine to leak out.
- Family history of prolapse: a woman may be predisposed to prolapse.
- Pelvic surgery or trauma: damage to the muscles or tissues supporting the bladder may occur.
- Spinal cord trauma resulting from a fall, nerve or disc problems, and osteoporosis: nerves and tissues that supply the urethra and pelvic muscles are damaged.
- Neurological diseases (multiple sclerosis, spina bifida, and stroke): damage to nerves and tissues may cause incontinence.
- Heavy lifting: the pressure in the abdomen causes the poorly supported bladder and urethra to sag into the vagina, and leakage occurs.
- Smoking: this activity may be associated with a heavy cough, which can result in strong abdominal pressure exerted on the poorly supported bladder and urethra.

Treatment

Stress incontinence may be treated in a variety of different ways, depending upon the severity of the problem. In some cases, a combination of treatments may be prescribed. Your doctor will consider the cause of your problem and your needs, preferences, and personal goals for your treatment before making a recommendation on how to proceed. The non-invasive treatments available for stress incontinence will be discussed in detail in chapter 10. These conservative, non-surgical treatments include:

- lifestyle changes: managing weight, dietary choices, and/or bladder training (timed voiding).

- physical therapy: mastering Kegel exercises, using various types of available vaginal weights, using portable biofeedback muscle monitors, and pelvic floor electrical stimulation.
- mechanical devices: using a pessary or continence guard.
- medications: selecting a medication that works with minimal uncomfortable side effects.

Surgery may be used to treat stress incontinence, because it can restore the bladder and the urethra to their normal positions. By preventing downward sag and by creating support, surgery can help those who experience discomfort and who are unsuccessful with the less invasive techniques available. Surgical options to relieve stress incontinence are discussed in chapter 11.

The Wrap-Up

- Forty to 50 percent of women with incontinence problems suffer from stress incontinence.
- Stress incontinence is caused by weakness of the pelvic muscles, the connective tissues, and/or nerves controlling the pelvic floor or the urethral sphincter. Leakage of urine occurs when abdominal pressure is increased by activities such as coughing, jumping, and laughing, and/or when the urethra must close but doesn't.
- Non-invasive, risk-free exercises can help reduce the severity of leakage in the majority of women who suffer from stress incontinence.
- Medication is not a preferred method of treatment. (Because there is no FDA-approved medication available in the U.S. to treat stress incontinence, medications are really not an option for U.S. consumers with this condition.)
- A wide range of surgical procedures is available to treat stress incontinence.

6

Diagnosis: Urge Incontinence

Chapter Highlights
- Urges and Surges
- Symptoms
- Causes
- Treatment
- The Wrap-Up

If your childhood was anything like mine, you learned the social graces of toilet training through bribes of pretty panties, a trip to the toy store, or promises of chocolate treats. Having progressed from diapers and rubber pants to adorable cartoon character underwear, those nasty, infrequent emergencies were curtailed by stops at "wee-wee trees" lining the Long Island Expressway or Grand Central Parkway. Mom was always well-prepared with a handy box of tissues for just such occasions. As adults, we have come to rely on the control that we learned so easily and so successfully years ago. Unfortunately, as we age, our bladder can become overactive, resulting in urge incontinence.

TECH TERMS

Urge incontinence refers to the frequent sensation that urination is imminent and that it cannot be postponed for more than a few minutes and, in some cases, may cause leakage of urine.

Urges and Surges

When the bladder is healthy, we are in control and can decide when and where to urinate. When, however, the urge is too strong and too overwhelming, we risk losing control and need to stop what we are doing to immediately find a bathroom.

Urge incontinence is the second most common type of incontinence. It affects people of all ages and the likelihood of experiencing it increases with age.

Urge incontinence, also referred to as an "overactive bladder," creates the sensation of a continuous, uncontrollable, and uncomfortable need to void, both during the day and at night (waking a person more than one or two times per night). Urgency and frequency alone, however, don't necessarily cause the leakage of urine, just a terribly annoying feeling of an intense desire to urinate—right now! A person with an overactive bladder, therefore, is not necessarily incontinent.

TECH TERMS

Sensory urgency is when the bladder feels very uncomfortably full but when there is no actual leakage of urine.

Urge incontinence is also referred to as:
- bladder instability
- unstable bladder
- spastic bladder
- uninhibited bladder
- irritable bladder
- detrusor instability

BELIEVE IT OR NOT

Want to compare notes? Want to talk about urgency and frequency? Until going for treatment, I voided at least twenty-five times a day. My panties were down more than they were up! I had to shop in warehouses to maintain an adequate supply of toilet paper. I even purchased a water-conserving toilet to save on my bill. Although my last drink for the evening was at my 6:30 p.m. dinner, I found myself in the bathroom at 7:05, 7:10, 7:15, 7:25, 7:40, 7:55, 8:05, and on and on until bedtime. There were times when the urge would come over me so quickly that I was in terrible pain, tears welling up in my eyes, and I could hardly make it to the bathroom in time.

If, without warning, you suddenly lose urine at the wrong time or place, you may be suffering from the most common, but definitely treatable, form of urge incontinence. Your bladder isn't properly controlling the body's reflex to release urine. The detrusor muscle (the muscle in the bladder wall) normally contracts at an appropriate time (when the bladder is full and you feel the urge to void). When your nervous system and/or this muscle malfunction due to instability or over-activity, they may squeeze involuntarily (without warning) and at the wrong time, resulting in the need to void more frequently than normal and causing unpredictable accidents. The leakage can be any amount, from a mere dribble to several ounces of urine.

TECH TERMS

Motor urgency or **detrusor instability** occurs when the detrusor muscle is unstable and causes involuntary contractions, leakage, or the immediate release of urine, creating a gushing feeling.

Do you have urge incontinence? Take this simple test:

1. Do you urinate more than eight or nine times per day?
2. Do you urinate more than two or three times per night? Does this urge wake you from a sound sleep?

3. Do you have trouble making it to the bathroom in time?
4. Do you lose urine on your way to the bathroom?
5. Does running water give you the urge to urinate?
6. Can you make it to your front door or to your bathroom but then lose urine before you reach the toilet?

If you answered yes to any of the above questions, there is a good chance that you are suffering from urge incontinence and would benefit from seeing a specialist such as a urogynecologist or a urologist.

BELIEVE IT OR NOT

On a short trip to my cousin's house, I was overcome with a persistent need to void. We were only five minutes from our destination, but I just couldn't hold it in another second. The pain was excruciating. It was nighttime, and highway lights and headlights illuminated the grassy area next to the road. I had no choice and had to relieve myself, covering up as best as I could, by the road's shoulder. Fortunately, I didn't get arrested for indecent exposure. The good news is that this would never happen to me today because I have learned how to prevent any more such embarrassing episodes.

Symptoms

The most prevalent symptom of urge incontinence is the sudden, unpredictable need or urge to urinate, often resulting in the loss of urine (to a lesser or greater degree) for no apparent reason whatsoever. You may feel the need to void, or void involuntarily when:

- you are sleeping.
- you drink water.
- you touch water (doing the dishes or the wash).
- you hear water running (when someone is doing the dishes).

- you are exposed to cold.
- you hurry home, and no sooner than you use your key (or garage door opener), you begin to leak urine. This last situation is commonly referred to as "key-in-lock" syndrome.

DOS AND DON'TS

When you really gotta go, whatever you do, **don't rush**!

- Rushing stimulates your bladder and makes you more acutely aware of just how full it is. This increases your urge to void.
- Rushing can make your bladder contract more forcefully and makes it more difficult to hold back urine leakage.
- Rushing exerts more downward pressure on your bladder, thereby pushing out urine.
- Rushing makes you lose your ability to focus on controlling the urge.

Do relax!

- Relaxing lessens the strong urge to void immediately, permitting you to take control.
- Relaxing allows you to concentrate on other activities, enabling you to wait longer before voiding.

If possible, sit for a moment until the spasm passes. The upward pressure from the chair on your pelvic muscles may help quiet your bladder temporarily, just long enough to buy you that extra minute or two you need to calmly walk to the bathroom.

Causes

For the great majority of women suffering from urge incontinence, there is no known cause. Occasionally, urge incontinence is the result of damage to the nerves of the bladder, the nervous system, or the bladder muscles. In other words, urge incontinence is caused by a bladder that misbehaves: the bladder muscles go into spasm or contract and squeeze at the wrong time or all the time, without warning, causing the urethra to close. Oftentimes, but not always, this causes leaks. When the bladder is inflamed (such as when there is a urinary tract infection, or less commonly, a bladder polyp, bladder tumor, or interstitial cystitis) or when the urethra doesn't completely close, urine remains in the bladder neck, causing that feeling of needing to void immediately. If a urinary tract infection (UTI) is the culprit, the leakage may be temporary. Once the infection is cured, the symptoms should disappear. If the urge remains, see your doctor, because something else may be causing those bladder spasms.

DOS AND DON'TS

Don't be embarrassed by urge incontinence. Incontinence can be improved in eight out of ten women. Fewer than half discuss the problem with their physicians; they allow the problem to go unnoticed and get out of control because they are reluctant to speak up.

The inability to prevent urination can be caused by any number of problems that fit into two main groups: detrusor instability and detrusor hyperreflexia.

Detrusor instability is the likely diagnosis when there is no neurological cause for involuntary bladder contractions. When the condition is successfully treated, symptoms normally disappear. Reasons for detrusor instability include:

- poor voiding habits (not voiding completely—this leaves the bladder always somewhat full and creates the sensation of constantly needing to urinate).
- infection of the urethra and/or bladder (urethritis [swelling of the urethra] and/or cystitis).
- bladder hypersensitivity (interstitial cystitis—this is associated with pain, frequency, and blood in the urine).
- chemical irritants (caffeine, artificial sweeteners, alcoholic beverages).
- obstruction of the urethra (from a growth such as a polyp in the bladder or from a kidney stone trying to pass).

- bladder cancer (rare, frequently associated with bloody urine).

Detrusor hyperreflexia occurs when there is a neurological cause for involuntary bladder contractions. Spasms result from damage to the spinal cord and nervous system. Reasons for hyperreflexia instability include:
- spina bifida (a birth defect of the spinal column).
- multiple sclerosis (a neurological disorder).
- stroke (also known as a cerebro-vascular accident).
- Parkinson's disease.
- spinal cord injury.
- pelvic trauma (from a motor vehicle accident, for example).

TECH TERMS

Urge incontinence is often **idiopathic**, a disease of unknown origin. "Key-in-lock" syndrome is an example of this.

Treatment

The main goal of any treatment program is to allow the patient to develop control of bladder contractions. Tools used to evaluate urge incontinence are the same as those used in the diagnosis of stress incontinence, already discussed in chapter 5. The treatments used to relieve urge incontinence are discussed in greater length in chapter 10. These treatments include:
- behavior modification: retraining the bladder.
- physical therapy: mastering Kegel exercises, using vaginal weights, and using portable biofeedback muscle monitors.
- medications: selecting a medication that works with minimal uncomfortable side effects.
- internal devices such as pessaries or InterStim therapy.

Surgery is generally not performed to relieve the symptoms of urge incontinence.

Do not let embarrassment, fear, or wrong information about incontinence prevent you from speaking to your doctor. The great majority of women suffering from urinary incontinence can be helped or completely cured. Call your physician and ask about a referral to a urogynecologist.

The Wrap-Up

- Urge incontinence occurs when there are spasms of the muscle in the bladder wall.
- The most common symptom of urge incontinence is the frequent, immediate need to void, often accompanied by leakage.
- Urge incontinence can have a non-neurological or a neurological cause.
- An experienced urogynecologist or urologist trained in specialized investigation such as urodynamic testing can evaluate your symptoms.
- Treatment includes behavioral therapy, physical therapy, medications, and/or devices.
- Surgery is generally not an option for urge incontinence.

7

Other Types of Urinary Incontinence

Chapter Highlights

- Transient versus Chronic Incontinence
- Overflow Incontinence
- Mixed Incontinence
- Functional Incontinence
- Reflex Incontinence
- Nocturia
- Giggle Incontinence
- Coital Incontinence
- Total Incontinence
- The Wrap-Up

Because I was spending so much time on the toilet, I bought myself a comfy, shiny, new white plastic toilet seat. And it occurred to me one evening, as I sat there emptying my bladder every five minutes on the dot, that my incontinence problem desperately required immediate medical attention. I knew that spending two hours or more reading a hundred pages of the bestseller *du jour* while trying to completely void was just not normal. This wasn't rocket science.

So off I trudged, totally embarrassed, humiliated, and uncomfortable, to my first urogynecologic appointment. The doctor and I chatted as she performed all the standard tests, which I failed miserably. I knew I wasn't going to hear that I was "fine." After all, how could I be normal and urinate thirty or more times a day? When the doctor recounted her findings, you could have knocked me off the plastic portable potty with a feather: my poor little body was plagued with two different types of incontinence. Before that moment, I had had no idea that there was more than one kind, and, truth be told, I didn't want to have to deal with two problems—wasn't just one enough?

The diagnosis left me distressed and disheartened but not without the will to fight my two battles to the finish. I conquered both stress and urge—a.k.a. mixed—incontinence in a very short period of time. So, take heart, sisters: if I could do it, so can you. All forms of incontinence can be successfully treated one way or another, though not every woman's incontinence may ultimately be resolved.

Transient versus Chronic Incontinence

The Agency for Health Care Policy and Research (AHCPR) lists two basic types of incontinence: transient (temporary, reversible, or acute) and chronic (long-term, persistent, but not necessarily permanent).

Transient incontinence is usually caused by an illness or a specific medical condition that is more or less short-lived and is, therefore, quickly remedied by appropriate treatment of the condition and disappearance of symptoms. It may develop as a result of:

- a stroke—when the brain, the spinal cord, the bladder, and the pelvic floor are not in good working order. It is also not unusual for people who have experienced a stroke to have episodes of chronic incontinence.
- surgery or after any illness that limits mobility, makes physical activity a challenge, or interferes with the mental awareness of the patient.
- bowel impaction or constipation, in which a large mass of hard stool lodges in the intestine or rectum. This may give a signal to the bladder that it's okay not to empty. The stool may also block or irritate the bladder by putting pressure on it, causing either incontinence or urine retention.

- depression. Doctors are investigating whether the same pathways that cause incontinence may also cause depression or if incontinence, itself, is just plain depressing.
- irritation or inflammation of the bladder (cystitis), the urethra (urethritis), or the vagina (vaginitis).
- the use of certain medications: diuretics (water pills that increase the output of urine and cause the bladder to fill more quickly); sleeping pills, muscle relaxants, sedatives, and alcohol that relax muscles to the point where the user becomes unaware of the need to urinate; decongestants, antihistamines, and nasal sprays that tighten the pelvic floor muscles, causing difficulty in voiding; antidepressants and narcotics that relax the bladder so that it doesn't contract properly.[47]
- a lack of estrogen, which may cause atrophic vaginitis/cystitis.
- a sluggish thyroid or diabetes.

Chronic incontinence develops slowly over a considerable amount of time and results from damage to, or abnormalities in, muscles and nerves, or from gradual changes to the bladder or urethra. Chronic incontinence persists after the medical condition or illness has been treated. The most common types of chronic incontinence are:

- stress incontinence
- urge incontinence
- overflow incontinence
- mixed incontinence
- functional incontinence
- reflex incontinence
- total incontinence

---

47 Urinary Incontinence Guideline Panel. March, 1992. Urinary incontinence in adults: clinical practice guidelines. Agency for Health Care Policy and Research, Public Health Service. Rockville (MD):U.S. Department of Health and Human Services.

Overflow Incontinence

Overflow incontinence occurs when you cannot fully empty your bladder when you urinate. This causes too much urine to collect in the bladder and its eventual overflow (because it is full), resulting in involuntary leakage or dribbling when the bladder exceeds its capacity. The bladder may not sufficiently empty as a result of:

- an underactive detrusor muscle that doesn't receive the necessary stimulation from the nervous system for the bladder to contract properly and eliminate enough urine. This muscle may be weak due to the use of certain drugs, fecal impaction, diabetes, spinal cord injury, radical pelvic surgery, spina bifida, back surgery, radical hysterectomy, overstretching of the bladder tissue, multiple sclerosis, and other medical conditions where coordination between the bladder and urethra is gradually lost.[48]

- a bladder outlet or urethral obstruction. Causes of obstructions in women are severe pelvic organ prolapse, in which an organ protrudes beyond the vaginal opening; scar tissue, which makes the urethra very narrow; spinal cord injury; and a large uterine fibroid, which may obstruct the urethra.

People who suffer from overflow incontinence feel as though their bladder is never empty; they have difficulties starting to urinate and then find that their stream is very weak and that they void very little. If untreated, overflow incontinence can lead to a bladder infection, due to the build-up of urine. Fortunately for us gals, overflow incontinence is uncommon in women.

TECH TERMS

An **atonic bladder** is one that doesn't contract or empty properly, possibly due to nerve damage. The bladder fills until it overflows with excess urine that dribbles out.

---

48   Newman DK. 1999. The Urinary Incontinence Sourcebook. McGraw Hill Education, p 67–68.

Mixed Incontinence

Mixed incontinence is generally a combination of the different types of the most prevalent conditions—stress, urge, and/or overflow—and usually requires a urodynamic workup for a proper diagnosis. For women, mixed incontinence generally refers to stress incontinence (there is leakage with strenuous physical activity) and urge incontinence (there is an overwhelming strong, uncontrollable urge to void immediately, and you can't make it to the bathroom on time). Mixed stress and urge incontinence is far more prevalent in older women than in older men. It is best treated by first correcting the anatomical problems causing the stress urinary incontinence. Generally speaking, the same anatomic deficiencies causing the stress incontinence may also be causing the symptoms of urge incontinence. When the stress incontinence is treated first, there is a better chance of repairing both problems.

In premenopausal women, stress incontinence is more prevalent than urge incontinence. By the time a woman is postmenopausal, however, this statistic is reversed. (Women are more likely to experience urge incontinence than men. As we reach our eighties, however, we become equally as likely to experience an overactive bladder.) Other types of incontinence, such as overflow incontinence, hold fairly steady as the lowest rate.

Functional Incontinence

People with functional incontinence have no problems with bladder function and control per se, but are unable to reach a bathroom in time due to the loss of mobility caused by:

- a physical disability (Parkinson's disease, arthritis, poor eyesight, etc.).
- decreased mental awareness (Alzheimer's).
- memory loss or confusion (unawareness of the urge to void, failure to remember the location of the bathroom).
- drugs that adversely affect alertness, responsiveness, wakefulness, mobility, and agility.
- inconvenient facilities (distant bathroom, inaccessibility for wheelchairs).

The elderly in acute care and long-term care facilities are those who suffer the most from functional incontinence.[49]

Q&A

Am I incontinent if there is blood in my urine?

Hematuria, or blood in the urine, almost always indicates an abnormality, unless atrophic vaginitis or cystitis (thinning of the vaginal and bladder tissues due to a lack of estrogen) is the culprit, or unless menstrual blood happens to accidentally get into the urine. Hematuria is generally caused by a bladder infection and is easily cured with the proper dosage of antibiotics. Blood in the urine, however, may also indicate more severe problems, such as bladder cancer or kidney cancer. It is not an indicator of incontinence. If you suspect blood in your urine, see a doctor immediately.

Reflex Incontinence

An individual loses bladder control when the nerves to the bladder malfunction or are severely damaged, resulting in a neurogenic bladder. The following conditions have neurological consequences that may cause a person to be relatively unaware of the need to urinate:

- stroke
- Parkinson's disease
- multiple sclerosis
- brain tumor
- spinal cord injury
- spina bifida
- diabetes
- herniated spinal discs
- severe trauma to the lower spine

---

49 Op. cit. Urinary Incontinence in Women. p 31.

TECH TERMS

A **neurogenic** bladder malfunctions due to damaged nerves associated with a neurological condition.

When a person suffers from reflex incontinence, involuntary bladder contractions occur, but the urge to urinate is completely absent. The normal micturition reflex (urination) is somehow interrupted: sphincter relaxation, bladder contraction, opening of the urethra, urine flow, and bladder contraction will cause unpredictable voiding when the bladder is full or otherwise stimulated (by cold air, for example), resulting in incontinence.

TECH TERMS

Nocturia refers to being awakened at night with the urge to urinate. **Nocturnal polyuria** refers to the excessive excretion of urine at night.

Nocturia

Most people sleep through the night or wake once, maybe twice, to urinate, and this is considered normal. Those who suffer from nocturia are roused from sleep several times, either because their kidneys produce more urine than their bladder can comfortably hold, or their bladder capacity is reduced. If you think nocturia is your problem, keep a voiding diary (see chapter 10), which will help you determine the time and the amount of urine you are voiding and will help rule out more serious medical conditions such as heart failure or bladder cancer.

If you produce more than one-third of your daily output of urine at night, you may suffer from nocturnal polyuria. Polyuria is uncommon. Its cure is pretty straightforward: rule out diabetes or more serious medical conditions and simply drink less fluid at night. Diuretics, that help rid your body of excess fluids, are sometimes suggested. Desmopressin (DDAVP), a drug that reduces urine production, is occasionally prescribed for use at bedtime, except for the elderly. Older people may experience relief if they elevate their feet for half an hour or so prior to bedtime.

If you produce more urine at night than during the day, you suffer from nocturnal detrusor overactivity (overactive bladder muscles at night). Behavior modification is the least invasive way to deal with this problem (see chapter 10). In the event that fails, medications such as DDAVP, diuretics, and anticholinergics and tricyclic antidepressants (Ditropan, Detrol) may be used to stop involuntary bladder contractions.

More bothersome than dangerous, nocturia can be successfully treated and is often curable. Doctors have recently been warned about possible memory impairment in the elderly taking anticholinergic medications for an extended period of time.

DOS AND DON'TS

Do see a doctor to ensure that your nocturia isn't caused by a serious medical condition.

Giggle Incontinence

Giggle incontinence goes far beyond the stress incontinence a person encounters when laughing too hard. Giggle incontinence occurs when a person who is laughing hysterically experiences an unexpected, unintentional, uncontrollable, and total emptying of the bladder. Giggle incontinence usually occurs in teenage girls who are otherwise continent. The cause of giggle incontinence remains undetermined, although unstable bladder contractions may be responsible. Giggle incontinence is almost always temporary.[50]

---

50   Weber, A., Walters, M., et al. Sexual function in women with uterovaginal prolapse and urinary incontinence. Obstet Gynecol 1995; 85:483–487.

BELIEVE IT OR NOT

I was a teenager with giggle incontinence. Every time I laughed, anything from a mild stream to a raging, flowing river would gush down my legs. And I laughed a lot. Can you imagine how mortifying that was? Even on the hottest days, I would carry a jacket, just in case someone told a joke and my bladder decided to let lose. Then I'd run home and hide my panties under my bed until they dried. Giggle incontinence disappears as mysteriously as it arrives. No one ever knew that this happened to me—not even my boyfriend, who'd be kissing me passionately as urine continued to drip down my concealed legs. I never told my parents. I just couldn't. And then one day, it was gone, but the memories of my humiliation remained.

Coital Incontinence

This is a tough one, ladies. Embarrassing as it may be, some of us leak urine during our most intimate moments with our lovers—during sex. Coital incontinence has been reported by as many as 30 percent of women surveyed in a urogynecology practice, with many reporting negative effects on their sex life and avoidance of sex.[51]

Q&A

Will incontinence or pelvic organ prolapse affect my sexuality?
Recent studies have shown that women with these problems experience the same amount of desire for intercourse, frequency of sexual activity, pain with intercourse, and satisfaction in their relationships as women without these conditions. Their overall sexuality remains unaffected. Women with severe prolapse, however,

---

51 Gray, T., Li, W., Campbell, P., Jha, S., & Radley, S. (2018). Evaluation of coital incontinence by electronic questionnaire: prevalence, associations and outcomes in women attending a urogynaecology clinic. *International urogynecology journal*, 29(7), 969-978.

may find intercourse to be difficult because of the sagging of their uterus into their vagina, or they may find themselves psychologically inhibited from performing.[52]

Yes, weak pelvic floor muscles, overactive bladder contractions, and/or incomplete bladder emptying may bring on an episode of stress incontinence. When a woman is aroused, even just slightly, the pelvic muscles may relax and cause her to leak. Penetration and the thrusting motion of intercourse may cause a woman to experience bladder contractions. Orgasm may result in such great involuntary relaxation of the bladder muscles that a woman will feel that the dam has burst. It's no wonder that coital incontinence inhibits many women from enjoying a rewarding sexual experience.

BELIEVE IT OR NOT

Fortunately for me, my husband is a very patient man. No, I never suffered from coital incontinence, but I must admit that I had my former gynecologist tutting and shaking his head when I explained that during sex I often had to stop several times to urinate. If my husband touched me the wrong way, I had to excuse myself to use the facilities. When we had intercourse, it was not uncommon for me to have to will away the impulse to stop and run to the bathroom. Yes, I made sure that I went to the bathroom before we started. That didn't seem to make a difference. The minute we got started, that miserable urge became apparent and drove me crazy. And yes, once we stopped, I usually had to make a rapid beeline for the potty again.

---

52   M. Nawal Lutfiyya1, Deepa K. Bhat2, Seema R. Gandhi3, Catherine Nguyen4, Vicki L. Weidenbacher-Hoper1 and Martin S. Lipsky1 A comparison of quality of care indicators in urban acute care hospitals and rural critical access hospitals in the United States. International Journal for Quality in Health Care 2007 19(3):141-149.

In the time it took to make love, I could have conceivably had to relieve myself four times! It should come as no surprise that after I got treatment for my mixed incontinence, my sex life greatly improved. Gone in a flash were those sudden urges to bolt to the toilet at the most inopportune of moments. I felt completely rejuvenated and free as a lark. And the Kegel exercises helped my body respond in a beautiful new way. I am living proof that incontinence and all of its underlying problems can be successfully treated.

According to the National Association for Continence, to successfully manage your incontinence during sex, you should do the following:

- Make sure that you empty your bladder and bowel prior to sex.
- Use a warm lubricating gel, such as KY or Astroglide.
- Avoid a position that may cause you to leak.
- Don't try to hide the problem. Share your concerns with your sexual partner.[53]

Total Incontinence

Total incontinence refers to a complete loss of bladder control. An individual with this type of incontinence constantly loses a small amount of urine and must wear a protective pad at all times. When and where urination will occur is totally out of that person's control.

Total incontinence may occur because the urethral sphincter muscle doesn't stay completely closed or there is a hole (fistula) in the bladder that empties into the vagina. The problem is rare and may result from injury during childbirth or from surgery in the bladder area.

---

53 Op. cit. The Urinary Incontinence Sourcebook. p 193.

TECH TERMS

Ectopic ureter refers to ureters (the tubes on the left and right that connect their respective kidneys with the bladder) that cause the leakage of urine because they are too close to the urethra or because they empty directly into the urethra or the vagina.

Total incontinence may be caused by the following:

- a bladder fistula. If a hole exists in the walls between the bladder and the vagina, for example, urine can leak from the bladder into the vagina and exit the body from the vagina. This is one type of fistula. There are many, and they are classified according to location.
- an injury to the urethra. The urethra can be injured as a result of an accident or surgery.
- an ectopic ureter. An ectopic ureter occurs when the ureters enter the bladder too closely to the urethra or when the ureters empty directly into the urethra or the vagina, resulting in urine leakage.

The Wrap-Up

- Transient incontinence is temporary and reversible.
- Chronic incontinence develops gradually over time and results from damage to, or abnormalities in, the urinary tract.
- Overflow incontinence occurs when the bladder does not empty sufficiently during urination, and excess urine dribbles out.
- Mixed incontinence is a combination of two or more different types of incontinence—in women, usually stress and urge incontinence.
- Functional incontinence generally strikes the elderly who have good bladder control but who are unable or unwilling to use toilet facilities due to physical disabilities or decreased mental awareness.
- Reflex incontinence affects those who are unaware of the need to urinate due to damaged nerves resulting from a neurological disorder.

- Nocturia occurs when an individual is awakened at night by the urge to urinate.
- Nocturnal polyuria is a condition in which an excessive amount of urine is excreted at night.
- Giggle incontinence is most prevalent among teenage girls who suddenly and uncontrollably lose urine when they laugh hysterically.
- Coital incontinence occurs when a woman loses urine during sexual intercourse.
- Total incontinence occurs when there is a complete loss of bladder control.

8

Oh No, Can't Go

Chapter Highlights
- Identifying the Problem
- Causes of Bladder Retention
- Treatments
- The Wrap-Up

I'm sure we've all experienced a bout of "bashful bladder" at one time or another in our lives. You know: you're in the ladies room, and there's a person in the next stall, perhaps even a friend, and the silence is deafening. You just can't seem to relax, because the thought of someone hearing you pee is simply too mortifying for words. After all, refined, sophisticated women don't make noise when they relieve themselves.

So what do you do when you really gotta go but just can't? Do you sit and pray that someone will finish quickly and flush the toilet several times or wash and blow-dry her hands? Do you plug your fingers in your ears, trying to trick your brain into thinking that the sounds of your urine hitting the water in the bowl will be inaudible? Or do you squeeze your eyes shut and push and strain, trying to force trickles out of your uncooperative bladder? I've polled my friends, and the consensus is that if you've done any of the above, you're normal!

Identifying the Problem
Did you know that you don't necessarily completely empty your bladder when you urinate? True urinary retention, however, is a condition in which the bladder

does not empty properly. If you suddenly retain a large volume of urine, the condition can be painful and will require medical intervention to prevent damage to the bladder. Chronic retention is generally caused by a gradually increasing obstruction to the bladder—from a mass such as a fibroid pressing on the urethra; from severe pelvic organ prolapse (POP), which may kink the urethra and block the urinary stream; or from a decrease in muscle power required to void.[54]

You can retain four to six ounces of urine in your bladder before voiding again without difficulty. If, however, you retain more than this amount, you may have a problem. A PVR test (postvoid residual urine volume [See chapter 4]) measures the amount of urine that remains in your bladder after you urinate. It can be performed either by catheterization or by a bladder ultrasound.

BELIEVE IT OR NOT

It was a beautiful, balmy spring Sunday: the sky was blue, the sun was shining, and the birds were singing. It was the perfect day for a trip to the Central Park Zoo. So my husband and I packed up the kids and drove into the city. We had spent two glorious hours feeding foul-smelling pellets to our favorite four-legged friends when we realized that it was time to grab a bite to eat. The others indulged in burgers and colas, while Mom, who still hadn't shed those excess pounds from her last pregnancy six years prior, suffered through a salad and a huge diet drink. We made a pit stop before our thirty-minute return trip home.

Just five minutes into the ride, however, I felt that nagging urge to urinate. And just as I had those feelings, we hit terrible, really awful traffic on the 59th Street Bridge. As our car screeched to a sudden halt, I knew I'd never be able to make it to the nearest bathroom, let alone home. And there were no "Port-a-Potties" on the bridge. The pain became so excruciating that there were tears in my eyes.

---

54   NAFC. Your Personal Guide to Bladder Health, p 19–20. [Updated July 2007].

I reached for my only alternative, an empty soda cup. I dove to the back of the car and squeezed the two kids into the front passenger's seat. Then I tried to go. And I tried and tried and tried. Despite the tremendous pressure being exerted by my bladder, I just couldn't relieve myself, couldn't get my urethra to relax to let the urine out. It was probably because I was so mortified to urinate in the car with my kids listening and watching. What would they think?

I kept pushing and straining, and gradually, after what seemed to be an eternity, the urine slowly trickled out of me. I couldn't empty myself completely, but I did manage to void enough so that I could make it home.

When urine remains in your bladder, it becomes a hospitable environment for bacteria to grow and multiply. This leaves you vulnerable to a urinary tract infection, which in turn causes you to urinate more frequently. If you do not empty your bladder completely, you may experience bladder infections, overflow incontinence, or even permanent damage to the bladder and kidneys. Your bladder may eventually stretch beyond its normal capacity, and eventually the overflow may just run out without a bladder contraction (See chapter 7). If you try to hold back the overflow instead of urinating, you run the risk of creating a pattern of poor voiding habits that may require medical intervention.

Q&A

What are the signs that I haven't completely emptied my bladder?
- You may feel that your bladder isn't empty.
- There may be abdominal swelling below your belly button.
- There may be abdominal tenderness or pain below your belly button.
- You may feel urgency and you may have to urinate frequently.
- You may have a weak urinary stream.

- You may have to strain, push, or bear down to empty your bladder.[55]

The National Association for Continence suggests the following tips for improving bladder emptying:

- Urinate on schedule even if you do not feel the urge to do so (every three to four hours).
- Try different positions to see which one gives you the best results.
- Try "double voiding": Go to the bathroom and urinate. Wait a minute. Try to urinate again. This technique will usually reduce the amount of urine left in your bladder.
- Talk to your healthcare provider about medications or self-catheterization.

BELIEVE IT OR NOT

Every aspiring New York City public school teacher must pass a written licensing exam and a physical. I passed the written test with flying colors, but the medical proved to be more difficult than I had anticipated. Now don't get me wrong. I was as healthy as a horse—everyone should be blessed with my gene pool. The problem I experienced was that when asked, I just couldn't give a urine sample. It wasn't that I had relieved myself recently and there was nothing left. On the contrary, my bladder was relatively full, but it wouldn't relax and let go.

I tried everything: I drank many glasses of water; I carefully lined the toilet seat with wads of toilet tissue so I'd remain comfortable; I asked someone to turn on the water; I plugged my fingers in my ears so that I could concentrate on my mission; and then I pushed and strained (with many well-needed breaks in between) for a period of three hours. Yes, that long, and I'm not exaggerating.

---

55 Conquering Bladder and Prostate Problems, The Authoritative Guide for Men and Women. Blaivas JG. New York: Perseus Press, 2001. .... p 24–26.

Finally I managed to eke out a few drops of the golden excretion—enough to satisfy the burly, impatient nurse who was now on overtime but who wouldn't allow me to leave without delivering my sample. It was a torturous experience and totally incomprehensible to me, because I was, in most other stressful situations, incontinent!

Causes of Bladder Retention

Urination is supposed to be an effortless, unconscious act. You get the urge, you find a comfortably clean toilet, and you empty your bladder. There's no straining, no pushing, no pain, no difficulty, no hesitancy. You just go. But for some of us it isn't that easy, and we may encounter the following voiding problems:

- Hesitancy: We can't get that stream started despite our best efforts. Maybe our stream is weak or dribbles. We use our abdominal muscles to strain and push to empty our bladder. Occasional hesitancy is normal, but when it becomes the norm, rather than the exception, there is a problem. Hesitancy may be caused by a urethral blockage (from a pelvic mass such as a fibroid); by a cystocele (a type of pelvic organ prolapse where the bladder sags into the vagina); by weak or non-existent bladder contractions (the bladder can lose its ability to contract as a result of stretching during childbirth, surgery, or by years of delaying the urge to void); or by poor learned voiding habits caused by an inability to relax while urinating.

- Intermittency: Our urine flow stops and starts, follows an "on-off" pattern, and is beyond our control. After we think we've finished, we drip or dribble, and we feel that we haven't completely emptied our bladder, even though only an insignificant amount of urine may be retained. Intermittency may be caused by impaired bladder contractions, by consciously or unconsciously alternately straining and relaxing while trying to urinate, or by a neurological condition caused by a spinal cord injury, herniated disc, multiple sclerosis, diabetes, or by an abnormal bladder muscle. A woman may dribble if urine gets lodged in the vagina or in a small pocket in the urethra (diverticulum) and is then forced out by gravity when she stands.

- Inability to urinate: We can't go at all. As hard as we try, nothing comes out despite an acute and painful urge to urinate. This can be caused by any of the above-mentioned conditions.

The two main causes of urinary retention are:
1. a urethral blockage (more prevalent in men).
2. impaired bladder contractions.[56] This happens when the bladder is not able (for whatever reason) to contract normally and in a way which would result in complete and thorough bladder emptying.

BELIEVE IT OR NOT

I am so jealous of my best friend, Chris. She never seems to go to the bathroom. We can be out all day, have a serious liquid lunch, go shopping, and then just hang out, and she rarely makes even one trip to the bathroom. At work, I never see her use the bathroom key, and she once confided in me that she only urinates about four times a day. For someone like me, whose panties are down more than they're up, this seemed like the ultimate in good fortune. I have learned, in my incontinence experiences, that there is a group of people, generally women, who void infrequently and have a large-capacity bladder and yet show no evidence of urethral obstruction or an impaired detrusor muscle. It may sound odd, but the condition is called "camel bladder," alluding to the desert animals known for their ability to retain a lot of water.

Other factors that contribute to urinary retention or voiding difficulties include the following:

---

56 Jackson SL, Weber AM, Hull TL, Mitchinson AR, Walters MD. 1997. Fecal incontinence in women with urinary incontinence and pelvic organ prolapse. Obstet Gynecol 89(3):423–7.

- Constipation, resulting from hard stool or stool impaction, puts pressure on the bladder and may cause urinary retention.
- Childbirth may cause trauma to the nerves, muscles, and delicate tissues of the pelvis, and urination may become painful. If you try to avoid the pain by not urinating, urinary retention may become a consequence.
- Fibroids (benign tumors that grow in the uterus) can cause obstruction at the neck of the bladder (where the urethra joins the bladder), making it difficult to empty completely.
- Urethral strictures can cause a reduction in the diameter of the urethra, which in turn causes a problem with the outflow of urine.
- Pelvic organ prolapse (POP) can kink the urethra, which may cause bladder obstruction.
- Drugs such as antidepressants, antipsychotics, narcotics, sedatives, muscle relaxants, antihistamines, decongestants, anticholinergics (drugs that stop involuntary bladder contractions), some nasal sprays, and over-the-counter cold remedies may be responsible for urine retention (due to a relaxed bladder or the overproduction of urine).
- Medical conditions involving nerve damage (diabetes, stroke, multiple sclerosis, etc.) may cause incomplete emptying of the bladder, resulting in urinary retention.

Q&A

What is a hyposensitive bladder?

A **hyposensitive bladder** is generally due to reduced nerve sensation that causes a person to lose the desire to urinate. Urine is retained, resulting in an overstretched bladder with a larger than normal capacity. At first, this condition is marked by underactive bladder/detrusor muscle function and incomplete bladder emptying. When left untreated, the bladder/detrusor muscle fails. Overflow incontinence may be the end result of this condition.

Treatments

How can you fix the problem of urine retention or voiding difficulty? Some solutions are really quite simple, especially if you are experiencing only a mild problem:

- Relax while urinating. Spread your knees apart and get comfortable. Try changing position: lean forward or move to one side or another so that the bladder neck gets repositioned enough to allow for better voiding. Try double voiding: Urinate. Wait a brief period of time and then try to urinate again.

- Check your list of medications with your doctor. Be sure to include all over-the-counter drugs as well as all herbal products. If urinary retention is a possible side effect of any of them, ask for a different medicine.

- Have fibroids or strictures checked and treated to reduce outflow obstructions.

- Correct pelvic organ/bladder prolapse through any of the non-invasive techniques suggested in chapter 10, or through surgery, discussed in chapter 11.

If the solution isn't simple, drugs (such as bethanechol) that help the bladder to contract, or drugs called alpha-blockers (such as terazosin) that relax the bladder neck area, can be prescribed. Drugs are prescribed when no major obstruction is found.

When the retention is temporary (before or after surgery) or permanent (as a result of nerve damage), self-intermittent catheterization may be the answer. You are in total control; you insert the catheter as needed. The use of the word "catheterization" can make a patient cringe because it conjures up notions of excruciating pain. This is not the case for those who must resort to this treatment. In fact, most find the process relatively painless, although somewhat irritating at the onset, and not as inconvenient as one might expect. If there is no other choice, catheterization is an invaluable option that allows an individual to lead a more or less normal life.

You can do this! It's a safe and simple procedure to learn. Here's how it works: a short-term-use catheter is a long, straight, thin, flexible latex or silicone tube that has a closed end with holes near the tip and an open end. Sometimes a new catheter is used each time the catheterization procedure is performed. Most healthcare providers, however, agree that this technique is not necessary and that cleaning the catheter well, inside and out, with soap and water after each use is sufficient. There is no need for surgical gloves or antiseptic solutions—just wash your hands thoroughly with soap and water. Grab a gob of lubricant and generously put it on the end with the two holes. Make sure to lubricate the length of the tube that will be inserted as you proceed. Remember, if you put too much goo on the tube before it is inserted, your fingers will slip, and you'll just get frustrated. The tube goes into your vaginal opening and through your urethra into your bladder.

Upon successful insertion, urine will start to flow. Pressing on your lower abdomen will help you to empty your bladder. When the flow has stopped, remove the catheter and clean it and put it in a sealed plastic bag in preparation for the next time. If you are diligent about hygiene, there is little risk of infection using this method.

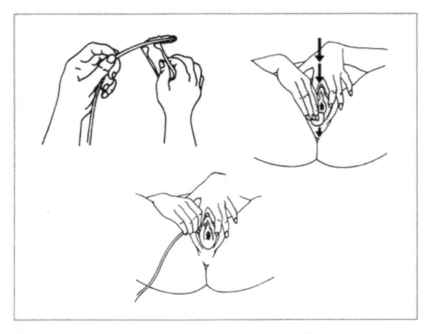

Self-catheterization in Women. Reprinted with permission. The Urinary Incontinence Sourcebook. McGraw Hill Education, Copyright 1999.

DOS AND DON'TS

Don't remove the catheter before the flow of urine has stopped, or you'll wind up spending a lot of time cleaning your bathroom floor.

A catheter for a woman is five inches long and may be straight or slightly curved. An olive tip catheter may enable a woman to more readily identify her urethra, because it is rounder, smoother, and a bit more rigid. The more rigid the catheter, the easier it will be to insert. Catheter guides are also available.

DOS AND DON'TS

Don't let too much urine accumulate in your bladder. Develop a schedule that enables you to catheterize yourself about four times a day and at bedtime. You may want to record how much urine you've drained from your bladder as well as the time. Over time, the amount drained may lessen, especially if you are able to void on your own as you progress. You may be surprised at how quickly your bladder remembers to contract to void. Your doctor may even tell you to throw the catheters away at some point. Wouldn't that be grand!

A Foley catheter, meant for long-term use, is comprised of a long, straight, thin, flexible latex or silicone tube. One end of the tube is closed but has two small holes and a small balloon; this end is inserted into the bladder. The open end is placed in a urine drainage bag. Smaller bags fit around the patient's waist, and larger versions fit around the patient's leg. The catheter is held in place when the balloon is inflated with a sterile solution.

A Foley catheter is used as a last resort for a person with urinary incontinence or retention that cannot be treated with medication, surgery, or intermittent self-catheterization. Generally older, surgical, or sick patients who can't care for themselves require this type of catheterization, which is avoided by medical practitioners whenever possible. To avoid medical complications, special care must be taken to change these catheters on a regular basis and to use a catheter that is large enough so that it doesn't become twisted or blocked. Insertion of a Foley catheter is usually performed by a healthcare provider under sterile conditions. These catheters do not fall out even when the patient performs normal everyday activities.

DOS AND DON'TS

Don't use a Foley catheter if it doesn't drain properly or if it is hard, brittle, or discolored.

The Wrap-Up
- Urinary retention can lead to overflow incontinence, to bladder infections, or to permanent damage to the bladder and kidneys.
- Hesitancy, intermittency, and the complete inability to urinate can be caused by a urethral blockage, impaired bladder contractions, poor voiding habits, or by nerve damage.
- Minimal urine retention can be treated with bladder training, drugs, or surgery.
- Intermittent self-catheterization is a safe, simple procedure that gives you total control over your bladder.
- A Foley catheter is used as a last resort, because if used improperly or for too long it can cause infection, kidney damage, incontinence, and bladder and kidney stones. It can also erode the urethra.
- Foley catheters are generally reserved for people who have had surgery or for those who are ill.

9

It's in the Rear, Dear

Chapter Highlights
- Identifying a Fecal Incontinence Problem
- Causes
- Screening
- Treatments
- Coping Mechanisms
- The Wrap-Up

Ladies, this is a very sensitive, touchy subject. While most of us will hesitantly admit to having experienced an incident or two of urinary incontinence, who among us would ever own up to a bout of fecal (bowel) incontinence? This is something that is just too humiliating to divulge, not to our closest friend and not to our healthcare provider.

Yet, I'm sure that since fecal incontinence is more prevalent in women, and since more than 5.5 million Americans suffer from fecal incontinence,[57] we've all got a story to tell that would raise some eyebrows.

So let's cut to the chase. Have you ever been ill and unable to control your bowels? Have you ever passed gas involuntarily at a most embarrassing moment? Have you ever passed gas and lost a little stool that left an ugly brown streak in those lily white panties? If you're being totally honest and you've answered yes to any of the above questions, you're a member of the club.

---

57 Johanson JF, Lafferty J. Jan., 1996. Epidemiology of fecal incontinence: the silent affliction. Am J Gastroenterol 91(1):33–6. [Medline].

Don't be ashamed, embarrassed, or humiliated. Take heart: one out of approximately fifty-three people in the United States has been afflicted with this condition, which affects between 7 and 18 percent of all women.[58] Let's discuss it in detail to remove the stigma and social isolation associated with it. Recognizing that fecal incontinence is a problem that can be managed and sometimes even cured is the first step toward giving a person back a large degree of control over her life.

Identifying a Fecal Incontinence Problem

Fecal incontinence is a medical condition that has many causes and varies in its severity: it can range from a small leakage of liquid or solid stool while passing gas to total loss of bowel control. Fecal incontinence refers to the inability to control one's bowels voluntarily, causing stool, liquid, or gas to leak unexpectedly and uncontrollably from the rectum. Many women who suffer from urinary incontinence also experience involuntary loss of stool or gas. Not surprisingly, many of the underlying causes of both types of incontinence are the same.

The following statistics demonstrate the widespread nature of this problem:

- According to the adult disposable diaper industry, over $12 billion is spent globally per year for adult diapers used to control urinary and fecal incontinence.[59]
- Fecal incontinence is the second leading reason for admission to long-term care facilities in the United States.[60]
- In one study, only 20 percent of patients suffering from bowel incontinence informed their doctors due to feelings of shame and embarrassment.[61]

---

58 Carrington, E. V., Scott, S. M., Bharucha, A., Mion, F., Remes-Troche, J. M., Malcolm, A., & Rao, S. S. (2018). Expert consensus document: advances in the evaluation of anorectal function. *Nature Reviews Gastroenterology & Hepatology*, 15(5), 309.

59 https://www.grandviewresearch.com/industry-analysis/adult-diapers-market

60 https://www.managedhealthcareconnect.com/article/5554

61 Nelson R, Norton N, Cautley E, Furner. Aug. 16, 1995. Community-based prevalence of anal incontinence. *JAMA* ; 274(7):559–61 [Medline].

- In a study reported in the Journal of the American Medical Association, 30 percent of individuals sixty-five years or older suffered from fecal incontinence, of whom 63 percent were women.[62]
- As a person gets older, the prevalence of fecal incontinence increases.[63]
- The long-term cost of fecal incontinence per patient is over $4,000 per year.[64]
- It is believed that fecal incontinence affects approximately 10 percent of all women.[65]
- Childbirth is considered the leading cause of fecal incontinence in women.[66]

Q&A

Who is at risk for developing fecal incontinence?

- Older people
- Those who experience urinary incontinence
- Women, due to complications of childbirth
- People with damaged nerves in the rectum and/or those who suffer from multiple sclerosis, spina bifida, diabetes, or late-stage Alzheimer's disease

Fecal (or anal) continence requires that certain conditions be met:

- The internal and external anal sphincter muscles must work together and contract to prevent stool from leaving the body at an inappropriate moment and to relax, allowing stool to leave at the proper time.
- A person must be able to sense in her rectum that it is time to go to the bathroom.

62   Op cit. Johanson.
63   Ibid. Johanson.
64   Xu, X., Menees, S. B., Zochowski, M. K., & Fenner, D. E. (2012). Economic cost of fecal incontinence. *Diseases of the Colon & Rectum*, 55(5), 586-598.
65   Seymour SD. emedicine [Internet].
66   www.fascrs.org/patients/disease-condition/fecal-incontinence-0

- The rectum must be able to stretch sufficiently to accommodate its stool content until a person can find the necessary facilities.
- A person must have the physical and mental ability to recognize and respond to her body's signals to defecate.

Causes

Fecal incontinence can have a wide range of causes, including the following:

- Constipation: Ironic as it may seem, constipation is one of the most common causes of fecal incontinence. Constipation causes large masses of dry, hard stool to become lodged or impacted in the rectum. The build-up of stool for days or weeks may cause watery stool that has collected behind the hardened mass to leak out. Chronic constipation can cause the rectal muscles to stretch and weaken to the point of not being able to retain stool in the rectum until a person can find a bathroom. The nerves of the anus and rectum will lose their ability to respond properly to the presence of stool in the rectum once they've lost their elasticity. Weak nerves and muscles don't work effectively.
- Diarrhea: The harder the stool, the easier it is to keep in the rectum. The loose, watery stools of diarrhea are harder to retain and can cause fecal incontinence or make it worse than normal. Even people who don't have fecal incontinence are prone to having an accident when they have diarrhea.
- Muscle damage: When an injury occurs to the ring-like anal internal and external sphincter muscles, located at the end of the rectum, fecal incontinence is inevitable. These muscles, responsible for keeping stool in the rectum, become weak and can't do their job if they are damaged. A woman's sphincter muscles may be damaged as a result of childbirth, especially if the baby is very large; if the doctor uses forceps to help deliver the baby; or if an episiotomy, a cut in the vaginal area to prevent it from tearing during birth, is performed. Women who experience

sphincter damage as a result of vaginal deliveries are at greater risk for developing fecal incontinence with each successive delivery.[67]

- Nerve damage: Damage to the nerves that control the anal sphincters or to the sensory nerves that sense that stool is in the rectum can result in fecal incontinence. Nerve damage can be caused by childbirth, a long-time habit of straining when defecating, stroke, spinal cord injury, and diseases that affect the nerves, such as diabetes and multiple sclerosis.

- Loss of rectal accommodation: Normally, the rectum stretches to hold and accommodate stool that accumulates until you can reach a bathroom. If the rectum becomes scarred or if rectal surgery, radiation treatments, or inflammatory bowel disease—such as Crohn's disease—have caused the rectal walls to stiffen and lose their elasticity, the rectum will not stretch as much as is needed, and excess stool will leak out. Inflammatory bowel disease also irritates the rectal walls so that they are unable to contain stool.

- Surgery: Hemorrhoid surgery, as well as other operations involving the anus and rectum, can damage the anal sphincters, causing fecal incontinence.

TECH TERMS

A **hemorrhoid** is an enlarged vein in the rectum or anus.

- Pelvic Floor Dysfunction: The following abnormalities to the pelvic floor can result in fecal incontinence:
  - decreased perception of rectal sensation
  - decreased anal canal pressures
  - decreased squeeze pressure of the anal canal
  - impaired anal sensation
  - a dropping down of the rectum (rectal prolapse)

---

67   MayoClinic.com. Fecal Incontinence.

- • protrusion of the rectum through the vagina (rectocele)
- • generalized weakness and sagging of the pelvic floor.
- • In women, a common cause of pelvic floor dysfunction is childbirth, and incontinence doesn't show up until the mid-forties or later. New mothers often hesitate to tell their doctors about their fecal incontinence problems. This is a mistake. The immediate repair of a torn anal sphincter muscle will help to prevent possible long-term complications.
- • Chronic laxative abuse: Relying on laxatives to maintain regularity can lead to fecal incontinence.
- • Age: As we get older, the muscles that provide support to our organs can weaken and lead to fecal incontinence.

Screening

Of course you'll have to visit a doctor for proper screening and diagnosis of fecal incontinence. Yes, you'll be asked a lot of embarrassing questions related to duration of fecal incontinence, type of incontinence experienced, frequency of episodes, type of stool lost, relevant surgeries, medications you use, dietary habits, number of and information about vaginal deliveries, etc., to determine if your problem can be easily remedied. You'll also have to submit your poor body to some uncomfortable exams and some mighty distasteful tests.

An initial evaluation by a healthcare provider will help determine the exact cause of fecal incontinence.

Your doctor will visually inspect your anus, your vagina, and the surrounding area in search of hemorrhoids, infections, skin tags, anal fissures, fistulae (holes), and scars that may indicate trauma to the region. To ascertain that there is no nerve damage, the perineal region (the area between the vagina and the rectum) may be poked with a pin or probe to ensure that the anal sphincter functions properly and that the anus moves as it should.

A digital rectal exam will be performed. That's where the doctor gloves up and inserts a lubricated finger into your rectum to determine the strength of your sphincter muscles, in order to ascertain if there is any rectal prolapse and to check for any abnormalities.[68] If rectal bleeding has been a symptom, or even if there has been chronic diarrhea or constipation (or any of these symptoms alone or in combination), a colonoscopy may be required in order to rule out something more serious, such as polyps (the cancerous and non-cancerous variety) or even colon cancer. Various diseases cause fecal incontinence, and these will be ruled out before further steps are taken.

Medical tests are also available to help pinpoint the cause of fecal incontinence:

- An anorectal ultrasound diagnostic imaging study allows the doctor to evaluate both the internal and external sphincters at work. A narrow, wand-like instrument that is attached to a computer and video screen is inserted into your anus and rectum. Sound waves bounce off your anus and rectum and produce pictures of them.

- Anal manometry checks the pressure of the rectum when it is resting or when it is squeezing and the sensitivity, capacity, and compliance of the rectum. This test involves inserting a narrow, flexible tube into your anus and rectum and then inflating a small balloon located at the tip of the tube.

- A proctography, also known as a defecography, shows the capacity of the rectum, how well it holds stool, and how well it can evacuate the stool. Liquid barium, used to make your rectum more visible on the x-rays that are taken by the doctor, is inserted to coat the walls of your rectum. This test can also be done using MRI.

- A proctosigmoidoscopy allows your doctor to look inside your rectum for signs of diseases or tumors, inflammation, or scar tissue that may be responsible for fecal incontinence. A long, thin tube with a tiny video camera attached to the end is inserted into your rectum and the last two feet of your colon, known as the sigmoid.

- An anal electromyography tests for nerve damage associated with an injury during childbirth. Tiny needle electrodes are inserted into the muscles surrounding your anus.[69]

---

68   Ibid.
69   Op cit. Seymour. Section 6.

BELIEVE IT OR NOT

We had just leased the car of our dreams, a beautiful, brand-new, baby blue Jaguar. When our friends Cindy and George suggested we drive into the city to catch a Broadway show and dinner, we eagerly jumped at the opportunity to take our new wheels out for their maiden voyage. The four of us piled in and off we went. The evening promised to be spectacular. Unfortunately, the show was just so-so and the restaurant we really wanted to eat in was packed. Undaunted, we settled for second best, and the animated dinner conversation more than made up for the mediocrity of the meal.

We were sipping our frothy cappuccinos and sharing a decadent chocolate dessert when Cindy's face suddenly grew pale and she bolted for the bathroom. She returned soon enough but made a mad dash again almost immediately, claiming that she wasn't feeling very well. No problem. We all knew what that felt like, and we patiently sat through four more hasty beelines to the ladies room. Finally, Cindy insisted that she felt much better, and we piled into the Jag for our trip home.

We were cruising along at sixty mph on the infamous Long Island Expressway when Cindy suddenly demanded that we pull over onto the shoulder. Just as she was exiting the car, her bowels exploded all over the back seat. The wonderful new-car aroma quickly dissipated. Instead, we were treated to the cloying, sickening smell of loose stool. Cindy cried. I cried. The men didn't know what to do. I learned an invaluable lesson that night: always keep a supply of towels in the trunk of your car.

But I digress. We drove home with the windows down despite the freezing weather, making every effort to control our constantly challenged gag reflexes. I could feel Cindy's humiliation and embarrassment, and I truly empathized with her. The next day I used an entire can of disinfectant and deodorant on the back seat of the car. I cleaned and prayed the entire time that I would never personally experience such humiliation.

Treatments

There are many effective treatments for fecal incontinence, such as physical therapy (including pelvic floor exercises), behavior modification, dietary changes, certain medications, or even surgery. In some cases and depending on the reason for the incontinence, one or several treatments may be chosen (either singly, sequentially, or in combination). You may be advised to seek care from or be referred to a gastroenterologist, a colorectal specialist, or another practitioner for the treatment of your particular condition.

What you eat and drink actually helps to determine the consistency of your body's solid waste material, or stool, as well as its transit time (speed at which this stool makes its trip) through your GI (gastrointestinal) tract. If you experience constipation on a regular basis (chronically), you may find some relief by increasing your intake of fluid and fiber (the non-constipating form) and by exercising regularly. Diarrhea may be improved by increasing your intake of high-fiber foods.

Foods that are rich in fiber include:

Breads, cereals, and beans	fiber
1/2 cup of black-eyed peas, cooked	4 grams
1/2 cup of kidney beans, cooked	5.7 grams
1/2 cup of lima beans, cooked	4.5 grams
Whole-grain cereal, cold	
1/2 cup of All-Bran	9.6 grams
3/4 cup of Total	2.4 grams
3/4 cup of Post Bran Flakes	5.3 grams
1 packet of whole-grain cereal, hot (oatmeal, Wheatena)	3 grams
•1 slice of whole-wheat or multigrain bread	1.7 grams

Fruits

1 medium apple	3.3 grams
1 medium peach	1.8 grams
1/2 cup of raspberries	4 grams
1 medium tangerine	1.9 grams

Vegetables

1 cup of acorn squash, raw	2.1 grams
1 medium stalk of broccoli, raw	3.9 grams
5 brussels sprouts, raw	3.6 grams
1 cup of cabbage, raw	2 grams
1 medium carrot, raw	1.8 grams
1 cup of cauliflower, raw	2.5 grams
1 cup of spinach, cooked	4.3 grams
1 cup of zucchini, raw	2 grams

Source: USDA/ARS Nutrient Data Laboratory Home Page. 2006. Release 19.

If an ounce of prevention is worth a pound of cure, you may want to try to manage fecal incontinence by doing the following:

- Keep a food diary in which you list what you eat, how much you eat, and when you have episodes of incontinence. If you see a pattern, you will be able to identify the foods that are giving you a problem. Try avoiding them to see if that makes a difference.
- Avoid foods that are known to cause diarrhea:
  - caffeine
  - cured or smoked meats
  - spicy foods
  - alcohol
  - fruits like apples, peaches, and pears
  - fatty and greasy foods
  - artificial sweeteners

- dairy products—milk, cheese, ice cream (for patients who are lactose intolerant)
- Eat smaller meals more frequently. Large amounts of food may cause bowel contractions that lead to incontinence.
- Don't eat and drink at the same time. Drinking liquids a half-hour before or after meals will help slow down the digestive and elimination process.
- Eat twenty to thirty grams of fiber per day in small doses to avoid diarrhea.
- In conjunction with a high-fiber diet, eat foods that bulk up your stool to slow down the emptying of your bowels:
  - bananas
  - rice
  - tapioca
  - bread
  - potatoes
  - applesauce
  - cheese
  - smooth peanut butter
  - yogurt
  - pasta
  - oatmeal
- Drink lots of water—one-half of your weight in ounces—daily to keep stools well-formed and to prevent constipation resulting from dehydration. Avoid caffeine, alcohol, milk, and carbonated beverages, which can trigger diarrhea. Learn to love water.
- Opt for an enema to empty the rectum prior to travel or an important business or social event. This is not recommended on a regular basis because the solutions used in enemas may rob the lower gastrointestinal tract of valuable bacteria. This may contribute, in the long run, to the return of constipation.

Medications may be recommended to control fecal incontinence based on the type and severity of the symptoms:

- Anti-diarrheal drugs or bulking agents (Citrucel, Metamucil, Fiberall, Hydrocil, Benefiber), which may be accompanied by a decrease in fluid intake, will reduce diarrhea by adding bulk to the stool and creating a more regular bowel pattern.
- Medications (loperamide) that inhibit bowel motility (the motion of your bowel) allow for increased absorption of water and, therefore, firmer stools.
- Mild laxatives (milk of magnesia) are prescribed to restore normal bowel movements when chronic constipation is to blame for incontinence.
- Stool softeners prevent stool from becoming impacted in the bowel.

Bowel training helps some people relearn how to control their bowels, either by strengthening their muscles or by training the bowels to empty at a specific time of day.

Bowel training through biofeedback is a safe, minimally invasive technique using auditory and visual feedback aimed at helping the patient to restore pelvic muscle strength. A pressure-sensitive sensor is placed in the vagina or rectum to measure contraction and relaxation of the anal sphincter around the sensor. By looking at the readout, the patient can determine whether or not these exercises are being performed correctly and whether progress is being made. Biofeedback has resulted in a "90% reduction in episodes of incontinence in more than 60% of patients."[63] The success of this method of treatment depends on the cause of fecal incontinence, how severe the muscle damage is, and the patient's ability to do the exercise correctly and to stick with it.

For some people, especially those whose fecal incontinence is caused by constipation, bowel training means learning to have bowel movements at a specific time during the day—after a meal, for example. It may take a while to develop a comfortable pattern, but the patient will then be able to better predict when she will have to defecate.

For some people, the only option for successful treatment of fecal incontinence is surgery. Several procedures are available, and the type of procedure used is based on the patient's history, physical exam findings, and the results of diagnostic evaluation. The goal in this type of surgery is to restore the anatomy to normal. The surgical options that are currently available include the following:

- Sphincteroplasty is surgery to repair a damaged or weakened anal sphincter. The long-term prognosis for this type of surgery is good (70–90 percent success rate) and the majority of patients feel there is improvement in their symptoms. Although the improvements first achieved by this surgery may diminish over time (with an approximately 50 percent failure rate by five years), the alternative to living with the debilitating and embarrassing condition of fecal incontinence favors surgical correction only if there is a defect in the sphincter and conservative management proves ineffective. Long-term outcomes are not encouraging.[70]

- Surgery is available to correct rectal prolapse. When a patient presents with chronic constipation, the ligaments to the rectum may have been stretched and may have lost their ability to hold the rectum in place. In this case, surgery may be needed to correct the rectal prolapse and to repair the anal sphincter muscle.

- In women, surgery to repair a protrusion of the rectum into the vaginal wall (rectocele) may be indicated.

- Hemorrhoids may prevent the anal sphincter from closing completely, causing fecal incontinence. A hemorrhoidectomy removes the hemorrhoid and the problem.

- Others require that a pacemaker-type device (the InterStim sacral nerve stimulator, also used for urge incontinence) be implanted to stimulate the muscle.

- A gracilis muscle transplant (graciloplasty), performed to restore muscle tone to the sphincter, involves replacing anal sphincter muscle with muscle from the patient's inner thigh. For some patients, moving the muscle and wrapping it around the anus provides continence.

- An artificial anal sphincter can be used to replace a damaged anal sphincter. This device, implanted around the anal canal, has a cuff that

70 Cheung, O., & Wald, A. (2004). The management of pelvic floor disorders. *Alimentary pharmacology & therapeutics*, 19(5), 481-495.

inflates to keep the sphincter shut until the patient is ready to defecate. A pump is used to deflate the cuff and to allow stool to pass. It reinflates automatically ten minutes later.[71]

- When severe fecal incontinence doesn't respond to the treatments listed above, a colostomy (ileostomy) is performed as a last resort. This surgery involves removing a portion of the bowel and attaching the remaining portion either to the anus (if it works properly) or to a hole in the abdomen called a stoma, through which stool leaves the body and is collected in a special bag. This procedure should be carefully considered only if fecal incontinence proves to cripple one's lifestyle. The cost of surgery, the use of anesthesia, and the lifelong obligation to wear a collective bag need to be evaluated before a final decision is made.

When fecal incontinence is the result of nerve damage, sacral nerve stimulation may be a viable option. The sacral nerves extend from the spinal cord to muscles in the pelvis. Direct electrical stimulation of the anorectal nerves, which regulate the sensation and strength of the rectal and anal sphincter muscles, is a treatment option for fecal incontinence. At first, each of the sacral nerves is studied to see which exerts the greatest effect. Then small needles are inserted in the lower bowel muscles, which receive stimulation from an external pulse generation. If the patient has a successful response to this procedure, a permanent pulse generator may be implanted in the abdomen.[72]

Q&A

How can I comfortably leave my house if I suffer from fecal incontinence?

Overcome your fear of having an accident by always being prepared. Here's what you have to do:

- Always use the toilet before you go out.

71 Op cit. MayoClinic.com.
72 http://www.hemorrhoid.net/fecalincon.php.

- If you doubt that you'll remain continent, wear a pad or disposable undergarment.
- Always have clean-up supplies and a change of clothing in your bag.
- Know where toilets are located so that you can get to them in a hurry if necessary.
- If you have frequent accidents, use oral fecal deodorants to increase your comfort level.[73]

Coping Mechanisms

Let's face it, besides being humiliating and embarrassing, fecal incontinence can prove to be downright uncomfortable. The skin surrounding the anus is very soft, delicate, and sensitive, and the stool that can come into contact with this skin as a result of constipation or diarrhea can lead to pain, itching, or sores that could require medical intervention. Here's what to do to relieve the discomfort and irritation:

- After a bowel movement, gently wash the area with water. If possible, wash in the shower with lukewarm water or soak in a bath. Pre-moistened, alcohol-free towelettes are a wonderful alternative for cleansing this area.
- Air dry the area thoroughly after washing. Don't have the time? Pat dry with a lint-free cloth or washcloth.
- Apply a moisture-barrier cream to the area after it has been thoroughly cleaned and dried. Ask your healthcare provider for a cream that is effective.

---

73 Subak LL, Quesenberry CP, Posner SF, Cattolica E, Soghikian K. 2002. The effect of behavioral therapy on urinary incontinence: a randomized controlled trial. Obstet Gynecol 100:72–8.

DOS AND DON'TS

Do not wash this area with soap, which can further dry out and irritate the skin. If toilet tissue is your choice, make sure it is moistened. Rubbing with dry paper will also cause more irritation.

Q&A

What is a moisture-barrier cream?
A **moisture-barrier cream** is a protective cream that helps prevent skin irritation from the skin's direct contact with stool.

- Use a barrier cream such as zinc oxide, which may provide relief from anal discomfort.
- Wear cotton underwear and loose clothing that allow the area to breathe. Tight clothes restrict air flow and cause skin irritation.
- Change soiled underwear immediately.
- If you use pads or disposable undergarments (specifically recommended for incontinence), make sure they have an absorbent wicking layer on top. This layer will protect the skin by pulling stool and moisture away from the skin and into the pad.

The Wrap-Up
- More than 5.5 million Americans suffer from fecal incontinence.
- Fecal incontinence is the inability to voluntarily control bowel movements; to discriminate between solid, liquid, and gas; and to put off defecation until a socially convenient time.
- Critical to anal continence are: properly functioning anal sphincter muscles, good rectal sensation, and adequate rectal accommodation.

- Fecal incontinence can be caused by any one of the following: constipation, diarrhea, muscle damage, nerve damage, loss of rectal accommodation, surgery, pelvic floor dysfunction, chronic laxative use, age.

- Tests to determine the cause of fecal incontinence include: anorectal ultrasound, anal manometry, proctography (defecography), proctosigmoidoscopy, and anal electromyography.

- Treatments for fecal incontinence vary from simple to more invasive. These treatments include: maintaining a healthy diet that contains the proper amount of fiber, using prescribed medications, practicing bowel training, undergoing surgery, and receiving sacral nerve stimulation.

- If you suffer from fecal incontinence, you can remain comfortable and regain control of your lifestyle by practicing good hygiene and by taking simple steps to avoid unnecessary embarrassment and humiliation.

- Fecal incontinence is not something to accept any more than urinary incontinence. If you have symptoms, seek out a specialist for a full evaluation.

10

Avoiding Surgery
Whenever Possible

Chapter Highlights
- Behavioral Therapy
- Keeping a Bladder Diary
- Bladder Training
- Kegels
- Cones and Weights
- Biofeedback Devices
- Mechanical Devices
- Medications
- Percutaneous Tibial Nerve Stimulation
- The Wrap-Up

I remember receiving a beautiful, pink diary for one of my birthdays, and every night I looked forward to writing down the most intimate details of my teen years. I stopped this practice, however, when I realized that my kid sister was ratting me out to my parents. I was a child of the '60s, so you can just imagine what her loose lips spewed forth to the old folks. No hiding place was safe in my house. As a person who grew up and enjoyed keeping records and taking notes, when I heard about keeping a bladder diary, I looked forward to making entries that I knew could help me find some relief.

As for doing bladder exercises, that posed no problem for me. Some of my friends consider me an exercise freak. I already did exercises for my poor old back, my tired eyes, and my unsure balance. Another set of exercises? Well, these were easier than most. They didn't burn many calories, but I could do them while watching my favorite TV show every evening or while riding in my car.

And as for pill popping, suffice it to say that I'd rather be popping French bonbons between my ruby red lips than a capsule or tablet. Besides, one multivitamin, two calcium pills, two flaxseed oil pills, two biotin pills, two fish oil pills, and one super-strength vitamin E pill are enough for one day! When I heard that I could avoid medication by doing biofeedback exercises, I was overjoyed. Also, because they do take some time commitment in order to be effective, they gave me an excuse to watch even more of my favorite shows. In the back of my mind, however, I knew that if I needed a pill, there were several on the market that could help me in my quest for continence.

I am proud to say that I achieved what I consider to be complete continence without even the slightest hassle. I have had excellent results by following simple, non-invasive protocols. You can, too. You've got to trust me on this one.

Behavioral Therapy

The main goal of any treatment program is to allow the patient to develop control of bladder contractions. Symptoms can be greatly alleviated through a multifaceted approach combining behavioral therapy with pharmacologic therapy or surgery.

Physical therapy is a wonderful, non-invasive approach to incontinence that requires relatively few office visits, because most bladder rehabilitation can be done at home. There are specific physical therapists trained in pelvic floor disorders. Regular check-ups with your physical therapist and with your doctor will ensure that you're on the right track and will allow for any needed adjustments to your individual treatment program. To have a successful physical therapy experience, you must be comfortable with your body, your sexuality, and your excretory functions, as the therapist may have to do some internal probing before determining the best physical therapy program for you.

Behavioral approaches to incontinence include lifestyle modifications, bladder training, and pelvic floor muscle rehabilitation. These therapies have virtually no adverse effects and are relatively inexpensive (especially when compared to surgery or the long-term cost of absorbent products) unless extensive or complex training is required. Incorporating behavioral changes into daily routines promotes feelings of self-control, and the idea of "natural" therapies is appealing to many women. Because these approaches are time-consuming, they require motivation and commitment if the therapy is going to be successful. It is essential to schedule follow-up visits in which the physical therapist, doctor, or other medical provider can monitor your progress and cheer you on.

Behavioral therapy focuses on retraining your brain to control your bladder, a "mind over bladder" approach. These techniques may help you become more aware of your pelvic floor and may suppress unwanted bladder contractions. The focus is on learning to observe exactly what things cause bothersome symptoms and then to concentrate on changing them. These techniques are safe, relatively easy, and non-invasive, and they have no side effects and are generally quite successful for a large number of women.

Keeping a Bladder Diary

A voiding diary is kept over a twenty-four-hour period for a day or two. Fluid intake and the frequency, timing, and volume of voids are recorded as well as the number and severity of incontinent episodes. Activities associated with incontinence should be noted. Here's a sample:

BLADDER DIARY

Name: _____ Date _____

INSTRUCTIONS

Column 1: Place an X each time you go to the bathroom to empty your bladder, or urinate.

Column 2: Each time you leak urine, use the following code to indicate the amount of urine.
   S = Slightly damp;
   M= Pad or underwear definitely wet, at least a tablespoon;
   L = Wet outer garments, large urine loss.

Column 3: Describe the activity you were performing at the time of leakage of urine (for example, sneezing, coughing, lifting, trying to get to the toilet).

Column 4: Describe the type of liquid intake (coffee, water, and so on) and estimate the amount (for example 1 cup).

Time	Column 1 Voided (X) in Toilet	Column 2 Urine Leakage S M L	Column 3 Activity with Leakage	Column 4 Liquid Intake
6–8 A.M.				
8–10 A.M.				
10 A.M.–noon				
noon–2 P.M.				
2–4 P.M.				
4–6 P.M.				
6–8 P.M.				
8–10 P.M.				
10 P.M.–12 A.M.				
overnight				

No. pads per day _____ Type: _____

COMMENTS: _____

Urine volume can be measured in a specially calibrated basin, creatively called a "hat," that is placed under the toilet seat.

Bladder Training

Bladder contractions are what we feel as the urge to urinate. The amount of urine in our bladders does not necessarily dictate when we feel the urge to void. With certain bladder conditions (urge incontinence, for example) this can occur with only a small amount of urine present in the bladder. This means that you may have learned to "need to void" more often than actually necessary. This learned behavior can also be unlearned. This is where bladder training comes in.

Bladder training is also known as timed voiding. Bladder retraining drills are very helpful and are usually the first line of therapy for an overactive bladder as well as for almost all types of urinary incontinence. This excellent treatment is completely safe and effective in improving or curing symptoms in nearly two-thirds of the women who need help.[74]

Bladder training teaches you to re-establish a healthy voiding pattern by gradually increasing the amount of your average void and by voiding on a schedule. When you void after increasingly longer intervals your bladder will readjust its pattern. This type of biofeedback technique can change your bladder's schedule for storing or emptying urine, in other words, "mind over bladder." These techniques are effective for urge, stress, or mixed incontinence and for overactive bladder.

This is when your voiding diary will come in very handy. By observing the patterns that appear in your chart, you can consciously plan to empty before you might otherwise leak. You can also learn to distract yourself and to refocus your attention until it is time to go. Your doctor or healthcare provider will look at your diary, will calculate the average interval at which you void, and will let you know what your target voiding interval is for your first month or so of training. You want to challenge your bladder gradually without overwhelming it.

Here's an example of how it works: Your goal may be to hold your urine for two to four hours (while you are awake). You may start by trying to hold urine for a one or two hour period of time. Once that time period is comfortable, it is then increased by fifteen to thirty minute intervals per week, or even by five to ten minutes per week or two to avoid any possibility of an accident.

---

74   Bo K, Talseth T. 1996. Long-term effect of pelvic floor muscle exercise 5 years after cessation of organized training. Obstet Gynecol 87:378–9.

Yes, it takes time, but you'll be surprised; you'll get there. This is a gradual process that corrects faulty, frequent voiding patterns that have become a habit; that increases the amount of urine the bladder can hold at one time; that teaches control of strong urges to urinate; and that may help reduce episodes of leakage from urge as well as from stress incontinence. When you can hold your urine for two to four hours while awake, you may find that your incontinence symptoms have improved.

Bladder training is a generally slow and deliberate process of educating your brain and your bladder to overcome past unhelpful habits. This involves a real partnership between you and your doctor (or nurse practitioner, physical therapist, and/or other healthcare provider). Be patient! It takes about six weeks to begin to see a positive change.[75]

If you hang in there, you'll be happy you did!

Here are the steps:

- Education: You must be given a clear and understandable explanation of your individual condition(s) and the procedures to be followed so that you can accomplish your goals.

- A voiding schedule: This may begin with two hour voiding intervals and increased to three to four hour intervals.

- Strategies to control urgency: These may include all or some of the following: pelvic floor exercises, deep breathing, distraction techniques (physical and mental), and relaxation exercises.

- Positive reinforcement from your doctor, nurse practitioner, and/or pelvic floor physical therapist: If you believe you will succeed, you will.

According to the National Association for Continence (NAFC), you can do the following to suppress the urge to urinate and to gain control over your bladder:

- Divert your attention from your bladder and focus on another area of your body. Concentrate on deep breathing rather than on your bladder. Continue to do so until the urge to void diminishes.

---

75   NAFC. Your Personal Guide to Bladder Health. p 18.

- Play word or number games to distract yourself so that you don't think about the urge to void.
- Concentrate on a task such as handiwork or letter writing.
- Give yourself repeated positive reinforcement about your ability to work through this problem.
- Focus on the muscles you want to relax and then perform your Kegels.[76]

Now, the chances are that you won't be able to completely reach your goal without further intervention. What follows are other things you'll probably need to do.

Kegels

The pelvic muscle exercises, first described by Dr. Arnold Kegel in the late 1940s, help tremendously with bladder control by strengthening and retraining the muscles of the pelvic floor and by improving the strength and timing of pelvic floor muscle contractions. Pelvic floor muscle exercises (PFME) are considered to be the cornerstone for all pelvic floor muscle rehabilitation programs to treat incontinence problems. Daily exercising of the pelvic floor muscles can improve and even prevent a weakened pelvic floor, prolapsed organs, and incontinence. These exercises are for young women too, and may even be helpful in preventing leakage during sports.[77]

Starting today, Kegels can be done for the rest of your life. Just as with any other voluntary muscle in your body, your pelvic floor muscles must be exercised on a regular basis to maintain their tone. Daily exercising (five sets of twenty, or ten sets of ten repetitions, for a total of eighty to one hundred contractions per day) can improve and even prevent urinary incontinence. They can be done while you are watching TV, driving a car, reading a book, or just about any activity, without anyone being any the wiser. They are easy to do, and most require no special equipment. Many women who have tried Kegel exercises feel

---

76   Wall LE, Davidson TG:1992. The role of muscular re-education by physical therapists in the diagnosis of genuine stress urinary incontinence. Obstet Gynecol Surg 47: 322–31.
77   Hay-Smith EJ, et al. 2001. Cochrane Database Syst Rev 1:CD001407.

that the exercises do not work, when, in fact, they have been doing the exercises incorrectly or for too short a period of time.

Women who have difficulty identifying their pelvic floor muscles can be referred to a specialist who can provide pelvic floor muscle training. Studies indicate that 20 percent of patients who practice pelvic floor muscle exercises (PFME) like Kegels have complete resolution of their symptoms, and 75 percent to 85 percent have significant improvement of symptoms.[78]

I'm going to share a secret with you that I learned from my urogynecological physical therapist: exercising your muscles by doing your Kegels will enhance your sex life, as well as that of your partner. So not only will your bouts with incontinence improve, but so will your love life. You can't go wrong. It really works. Trust me.

How to do a Kegel:

Quick Flicks

Tighten and then relax the pelvic muscles as quickly as possible. To identify these muscles, just keep in mind that they are the ones you need to stop a stream of urine or hold back gas. Pull in and up and squeeze those muscles (both the rectal and vaginal muscles) while concentrating on not tightening your buttocks or abdomen. Contract for one second and then release rapidly and relax for two seconds. Do between ten to twenty repetitions per day. Once you build up to a total of eighty to one hundred contractions a day, you're doing a great job. Remember, do not strain, bear down, hold your breath, or contract other muscles in your body when doing a quick flick.

Another way to identify the pelvic floor muscles is to try to stop the stream of urine when you urinate. Only use this stop-and-start method to identify the muscles and not to perform Kegel exercises on a regular basis, because it may lead to bladder infections.

If you have difficulty locating the muscles by yourself, vaginal cones, vaginal weights, and biofeedback machines can help you perform the pelvic floor muscle contractions correctly.

---

78   Lukban JC, et al. 2006. Int Urolgynecol J [Internet].

You can also try this trick: insert a tampon into your vagina and lie down on your back with your knees bent slightly. Try to prevent removal of the tampon by tightening the vagina as you pull gently on the tampon string. The muscles that you're using to prevent the tampon from come out are your "Kegel muscles!"

The "pelvic block" is used to prevent leakage prior to a cough or sneeze. It is started deliberately before the stress of the cough or sneeze (if you know it's coming!) and is held longer than a quick flick (until the stress is over). It's like a quick flick with an extension. It is not as successful for repetitive lifting, for instance, if you are lifting weights over and over. Unlike the "slow and easy" pelvic floor muscle exercise described next, which improves muscle tone over the long-term, the pelvic block is an intentional, fast, strong pelvic muscles contraction used before and during activity that causes you to leak. The key to success with this maneuver is to remember to start the "quick flick" before the cough or sneeze and not after it has started to occur.

Slow and Easy

This type of contraction helps you keep your pelvic floor strong over the long-term. Here's how it's done: tighten your pelvic muscles (as described above), hold for a count of five to ten seconds, and then relax for a count of ten to twenty seconds. As long as you relax for twice as long as you've contracted, you are on the right track. Again, these can be done sitting, standing, or lying down. These exercises really work, so hang in there!

DOS AND DON'TS

Don't overdo your Kegels, because this could result in doing more harm than good. Think of this as an exercise program for your pelvis. Just as you wouldn't over-exercise any other muscle in your body, don't over-exercise your pelvic muscle. Do not try to stop your stream of urine or do a Kegel while urinating (unless it's to help you identify your pelvic floor muscles)! This may damage your urethra.

Cones and Weights

Special cones or vaginal weights can also be used to strengthen pelvic muscles and reduce unwanted bladder contractions. These look like smooth, white vaginal suppositories or tampons and vary in weight from less than one ounce to a few ounces, even though they are all the same size, shape, and volume. You begin by inserting the heaviest weight (that won't fall out) that your vagina can hold. You do this for a period of fifteen minutes, twice a day. Your pelvic muscles will naturally grip the cone in a tight contraction so that the cone will not fall out. This is like an extension of Kegel exercises, just with the vaginal cone/weight acting as a "gentle reminder." You can also practice your quick flicks and pelvic blocks with the cone in place.

At first, you will be instructed to walk gently, with the cones or weights in place, for the entire time period of the training session. As you progress, you will then be instructed to cough, bend, climb stairs, and jump up and down while keeping the cones in place. Once you have been able to use this cone for fifteen to twenty minutes per day, twice daily (usually after at least one month), you will be asked to progress to the next heaviest cone, until you are working with the maximum weight. Over a period of time, the pelvic muscles will strengthen, and the symptoms of urge (as well as stress) incontinence may actually decrease.

Vaginal cones are cool, smooth, easily insertable, and have a nice large loop (that's a thread of permanent nylon-like fishing line) for quick removal. No need to agonize; unlike with a tampon, you never have to worry about losing that string inside you or forgetting to remove it. The cone itself just slips out so easily that, at first, it's kind of frustrating trying not to let it plop out of you. I started by using mine in the shower and then, besides singing, I'd bend and jump and do calisthenics, trying to work my way up to the highest weight. Sometimes, when no one else was around, I'd go up and down the stairs pulling my muscles as hard as I could to keep the cone from succumbing to the effects of gravity.

I got there. So can you.

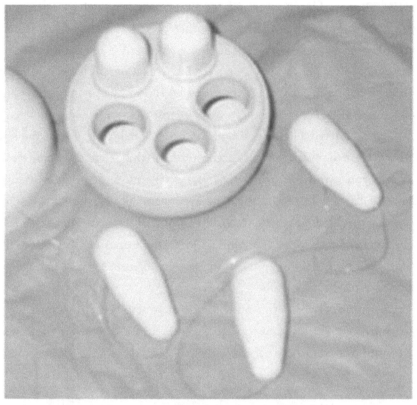

A Set of Vaginal Cones. Reprinted with permission. J.M. Rabin, MD

Another type of cone-like device to help you do your Kegels is the Colpexin Sphere. Colpexin has also been shown to be effective in reducing urinary leakage and prolapse and in strengthening the pelvic floor muscles. The smallest sphere is usually tried first until a good fit is found. Once it is in place, pelvic muscle exercises may be performed.[79]

Biofeedback Devices

Biofeedback devices provide immediate information about your pelvic floor baseline tone and your pelvic floor strength with a contraction. Units may be stationary (for use in your doctor's office) or portable (for your home training

79 JAMA. May 12, 1989. 261(18):2688.

program). The portable units are available for rent or sale though your practitioner. Biofeedback units (whether used in the office or at home) use visual computer graphic displays or auditory signals to show how well you are contracting and relaxing your pelvic floor muscles on a moment-to-moment basis. You must do all the work yourself, but you are rewarded by seeing how many lights you can turn on, depending on the strength of your muscles. In general, the feedback that you receive may be lights that light up or bells that ring. This is the reward that you get for the work you just accomplished (the pelvic floor contraction). The harder you work, the greater the reward (the more or brighter the lights, louder the bells) and, hopefully, the more improvement you'll notice. Most newer biofeedback machines have an entertaining group of lights or interesting sounds as your reward for all your hard work. Once you've mastered the biofeedback machine, your body will respond automatically and correctly in situations where incontinence might prove to be a problem.

Vaginal probes (which you purchase from your physical therapist for your own personal use) are easy and comfortable to insert and remove. They give you more control over your pelvic floor.

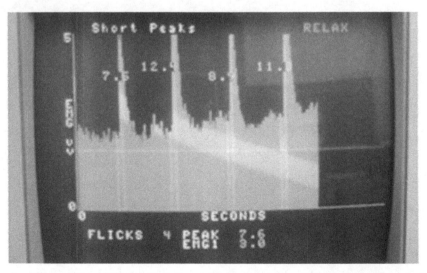

Display of Actual Kegel "Quick Flicks" on a Biofeedback Monitor. Used with permission.
Marilyn Freedman, P.T., B.C.I.A.-P.M.D.B., Louise E. Marks, M.S.,O.T.R.

According to the Journal of the American Medical Association: "When used in patients with stress and/or urge incontinence, biofeedback has been shown to result in complete control of incontinence in approximately 20% to 25% of patients and to provide important improvement in another 30%."[80]

Functional Electrical Stimulation

Electrical stimulation (enhanced biofeedback) is added to biofeedback when biofeedback techniques need a gentle push. Electrical stimulation occurs when a small instrument is inserted into your vagina. You will feel a tiny hum or a pulse that causes the pelvic muscles to contract for you. It doesn't hurt (all you can feel is a lifting or tightening sensation) and, trust me, it works! And no, it doesn't feel anything like a vibrator. This is a useful technique because, combined with biofeedback therapy, it allows you to locate and contract your pelvic floor muscles. Electrical stimulation is not for you if you have a pacemaker, are pregnant, have a pelvic or bladder infection, or are experiencing any bleeding. Make sure to let your physical therapist know if you have any of these conditions before starting this therapy.

Mechanical Devices

Pelvic organ prolapse can be corrected by surgery, but why opt for that solution when a non-surgical measure is available? A mechanical device known as a pessary (from the Greek word *pessos*, meaning "oval stone") may be inserted into the vagina to ensure support of the pelvic organs in cases of prolapse. Avoiding the knife, if possible, seems to be the best way to go, especially given the fact that operations are expensive. A pessary costs about one hundred dollars (depending upon your insurance coverage) and is covered by most medical insurance plans. Remember, in most cases, surgery is elective and does not necessarily have to be the first line of treatment.

Pessaries have been in existence since Classical Greek and Roman times, when creative medical practitioners inserted pomegranates, potatoes, string balls, sponges, and the like into the vagina to support sagging pelvic organs.

---

80 Burgio KL, Locher JL, Goode PS, et al. 1998. Behavioral vs drug treatment for urge urinary incontinence in older women: a randomized controlled trial. JAMA 280:1995–2000.

Fortunately, plastics became popular in the 1950s, and today most pessaries are produced from sophisticated silicone and other materials. Over the years, pessaries were used to treat a misplaced or tipped uterus, a weak cervix, and menstrual irregularities in addition to pelvic organ prolapse. Today they are used mainly for problems of prolapse and incontinence when support is needed for weak tissues and organs. These are especially popular for elderly women who, for medical reasons, may not be surgical candidates.

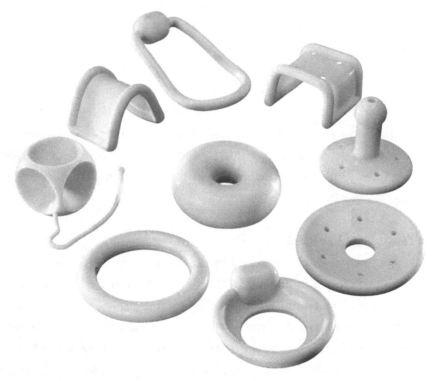

Various Types of Available Pessaries. Used with permission. Cooper Surgical-Milex, Inc.

Over twenty different types of pessaries are in use today. They are available in a variety of shapes or types, and each type comes in various sizes. One popular type, the ring pessary, resembles a contraceptive diaphragm and has a hard outside rim. Pessaries are made of different materials, but those made of silicone are preferred because they last longer and don't absorb secretions and odors readily. Silicone pessaries can be sterilized without melting.

A pessary is a very personal item, and if you choose to use one, you must be evaluated by a medical practitioner and then fitted individually for it to do its job effectively. If you are considering using a pessary, you may want to ask yourself these questions before proceeding further:

- Will it bother me to have something inside my vagina at all times?
- Will I remember to take care of the pessary by cleaning it daily, if necessary, and by returning for all the necessary follow-up visits?
- Do I understand that a pessary needs a routine cleaning by my medical practitioner?
- Can I accept that the pessary acts as a Band-Aid rather than a cure for the problem?
- Do I understand the side effects and complications that may result from the use of a pessary?
- Can I accept that I may get bladder and vaginal infections from using a pessary?
- Can I accept that if certain side effects and complications exist, I may not be a candidate for a pessary and that I should look for other remedies?
- Do I understand that fitting a pessary is sometimes a difficult endeavor and that I may have to go back to have the fit corrected?
- Am I comfortable inserting and removing the pessary?
- Will the use of a pessary inhibit my sex life?

Q&A

Can I engage in sex while I'm wearing a pessary?
You may wear a ring pessary during intercourse if you are comfortable. It is recommended that all other pessaries be removed prior to intercourse.

Here are some different types of pessaries and their uses:

- The **ring without support** is used to lift internal pelvic organs such as the bladder and rectum where support of the cervix and uterus is sufficient and additional support in this area is not needed.

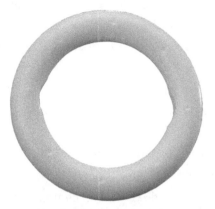

Ring without Support. Used with permission. Cooper Surgical-Milex, Inc.

- The **ring with support** is used for mild uterine prolapse complicated by a mild cystocele (dropping of the bladder into the vagina) and/or rectocele (dropping of the rectum into the vagina).

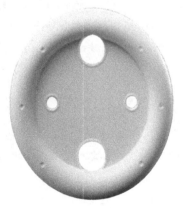

Ring with Support. Used with permission. Cooper Surgical-Milex, Inc.

- The supportive **Shaatz** pessary may also be used for mild uterine prolapse complicated by a mild cystocele and/or rectocele.

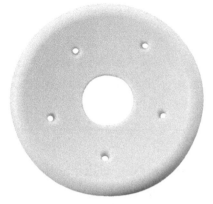

The Shaatz Pessary. Used with permission. Cooper Surgical-Milex, Inc.

- The supportive **Regula** pessary, with a unique design that helps to prevent expulsion, is also indicated for mild to moderate uterine prolapse.

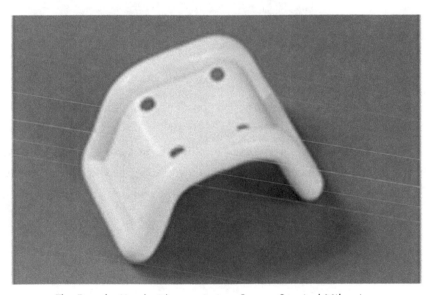

The Regula. Used with permission. Cooper Surgical-Milex, Inc.

TECH TERMS

Procidentia refers to one of the most severe forms of prolapse, in which the uterus sags to a point where it is actually dropping outside of the body.

For more severe prolapse, such as procidentia, the following pessaries are used:
- The **donut** pessary is very effective in supporting severe prolapse.

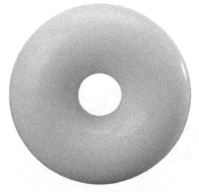

Donut Pessary. Used with permission. Cooper Surgical-Milex, Inc.

- The **Gellhorn** pessary comes in silicone, in both a rigid and flexible form, and is one of the most popular pessaries used in the treatment of severe prolapse. It offers excellent support and drainage of secretions.

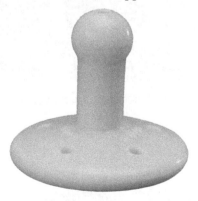

The Gellhorn Pessary. Used with permission. Cooper Surgical-Milex, Inc.

- The space-filling **Inflatoball** pessary, made of latex rubber, works well for moderate to severe prolapse. Drawbacks include the fact that it must be removed daily, over-inflation will cause a bulge, and it requires tremendous skill to attach, to inflate, and to detach it without losing air. Those with an allergy to latex must avoid the **Inflatoball** pessary.

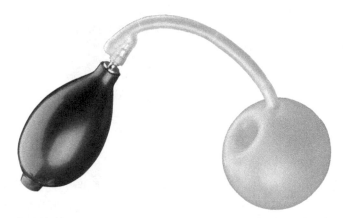

The Inflatoball Pessary. Used with permission. Cooper Surgical-Milex, Inc.

- The **cube**, especially the tandem-cube, is used as a last resort only when other pessaries will not be retained. It is kept in place by suction and can cause vaginal erosions if not removed properly. It should not be used in patients with uncontrolled diabetes because it may cause ulcers and other more severe medical conditions.

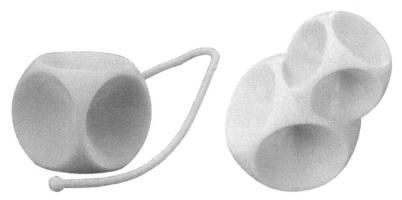

The Cube Pessary (left) and the Tandem Cube (right). Both used with permission. Cooper Surgical-Milex, Inc.

- The **Gehrung's** flexibility and adaptability in raising the pelvic floor make it an excellent choice in the treatment of prolapse.

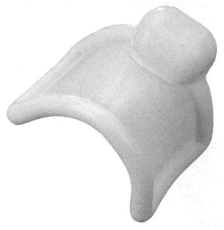

Gehrung Pessary with Knob. Used with permission. Cooper Surgical-Milex, Inc.

Other pessaries

Some other pessaries include the **Hodge, Risser, Smith, Incontinence Dish/ring**, and pessaries with knobs. Some suggest that the knob pessaries (see **Gehrung** with knob) help reduce leakage by compressing the urethra. The knob may rotate and compress other delicate structures.

Q&A

Are there any complications associated with the use of a pessary?
Most complications are minor and correctible. A common problem is improper fit. Irritation, erosion, ulceration of the vagina, and/or vaginal fistulas (holes in the vaginal walls) can also occur with improper fit, care, and/or maintenance of the pessary. Other side effects include back pain, vaginal odor, white vaginal discharge (leucorrhea) caused by the presence of a foreign object in the vagina, bleeding, pain, and urinary or stool retention.

If the pessary is forgotten for a long period of time (generally over years), it may cause vaginal cancer or erode through the vagina into the pelvis.

Pessaries must be properly fitted and cared for, which takes a bit of patience. Fitting the pessary is truly more of an art than a science and requires some trial, error, and experience on the part of the medical provider. If the pessary doesn't fit properly, complications can arise. If it's too small, it can move and/or fall out. If it's too large, it most certainly will be quite uncomfortable and can irritate the vagina and obstruct the passage of urine. The least bulky device that relieves your symptoms will be selected.

Q&A

Are there any products available to reduce irritation and discomfort?
You can use **Trimo San**, an antibacterial gel and lubricant. It maintains a healthy low vaginal pH level and reduces odor-causing bacterial growth. **Trimo San** is used as follows: one-half applicator inserted three times during the first week of use and then twice a week thereafter. Alternatively, low-dose vaginal estrogen can be used. Ask your doctor or nurse practitioner for the best program to fit your needs.

Here is what you can expect if you opt for a pessary:
- The doctor will determine the type of prolapse you have and its severity.
- The proper type of pessary will then be selected.
- A digital exam will be performed to determine the size needed.
- The pessary will be inserted. Ask to see it before it's inserted so you know what is being put inside your body.
- You will be asked to bear down, stand, sit, walk, and use the toilet. You may be asked to feel the pessary (the sensation of the pessary as you

bear down and/or the physical feeling as you reach into your vagina and touch the pessary with one or two fingers) while you are bearing down. If not, ask to do so.

- The doctor will re-examine you while standing to ensure that the pessary does not shift too much.

DOS AND DON'TS

If you are going for an MRI (magnetic resonance imagining), remove any pessary containing a metal cord prior to the procedure, as the magnetism rotating around you will rip the metal right out of your body (not a pretty thought!).

Once you've had a pessary inserted, make sure to return to your medical practitioner for follow-up care that may include any or all of the following:

- A follow-up exam within two weeks.
- Return visits every two to three weeks.

During an exam, the doctor will:

- Ask you if you are urinating and defecating without any new problems since the pessary was inserted.
- Answer any of your questions.
- Remove the pessary.
- Clean the pessary.
- Perform a vaginal exam including a vaginal rinse.
- Reinsert the pessary if there are no contraindications.

Q&A

Are there any women who shouldn't use a pessary?
Yes. Women with the following conditions should not use a pessary and should find another way to remain continent:

- a vaginal infection.

- recent vaginal surgery.
- a previous serious condition as a result of pessary use, such as vaginal cancer.

Pessaries will have the best results when the delicate vaginal tissues are well-estrogenized. If you are past menopause, ask your doctor about using a small amount of an estrogen-based vaginal cream on a regular basis. This may make pessary use more comfortable. If estrogen is not for you, ask your doctor to recommend a good lubricant, such as **Trimo San**. Look for lubricants that are non-irritating and comfortable to the user, water soluble, unscented, and of a pleasant consistency.

Most women can insert and remove the pessary at will, while others cannot. To insert a pessary by yourself, do the following:

- Either lubricate the pessary or your vagina with the lubricant of your choice.
- Place the pessary high and to the back of your vagina. (If this is not comfortable, remove and reinsert.) Don't repeat this cycle more than once without consulting your practitioner.

A pessary can remain inside your body (except for the **cube and Inflatoball**, which must be removed every day) for up to one month, as long as you are careful to remove and clean it after that period of time. Shorter intervals (one week) are generally better for reducing the chance of vaginal infection and for allowing the user to deal with vaginal secretions that naturally build up with time. Make a schedule that works best for you.

To remove the pessary yourself, do the following:

- Empty your bladder.
- Get into a comfortable position (lying down or sitting, even standing).
- Reach with your fingers up into the vagina, find the pessary, and gently glide it out in a downward direction. You may want to push a bit as if you're defecating, which will bring the pessary closer to your fingers.

- Finally, wash the pessary with gentle soap and warm water. Dry it off and re-insert it once you're ready.

Q&A

Why treat prolapse and incontinence with a pessary?
There are three good reasons:

1. The pessary is a good device that has stood the test of time. It reduces prolapse and thus may make you more comfortable (generally less prolapse leads to greater comfort) faster than other therapies. Its effect may be felt immediately, but in many cases may take several days to get used to.
2. Pessaries will help you see how you feel with your pelvic organs in place so that you can decide when and if you want or need surgery on your own time schedule. A pessary may be removed at any time.
3. Using a pessary instead of a medication saves money and avoids side effects such as dry mouth, constipation, and serious drug interactions.

Medications

Medications for overactive bladder and urge incontinence help relax your bladder, thereby controlling its contractions so that it can hold more urine and for longer intervals. Non-drug therapy is recommended as a first-line treatment for overactive bladder. Pelvic floor muscle exercises and bladder training are time-tested and can be more effective than medication.[81] Also, less is more. Your doctor should prescribe the lowest dose that works for you

Medications for stress incontinence tighten muscles at the neck of the bladder and urethra, thus preventing leakage. Although medication can be used to treat stress incontinence, there is currently no medication in the United

---

81   Kalant H, Grant D, Mitchell J. 2006. Principles of Medical Pharmacology,Seventh ed. Part 2, Autonomic Nervous System. Saunders.

States approved to treat this condition. Drugs that artificially help the urethral sphincter stay sufficiently closed (drugs found in common cold decongestants and allergy remedies) provide some relief but may produce uncomfortable side effects. No convincing medical evidence exists supporting the use of these drugs for this condition.

Beware! Drugs are used to relieve symptoms and not to provide a cure. You don't want to become dependent upon them. Try other methods of bladder control before resorting to medication. You wouldn't want to have to pop pills indefinitely! On the other hand, drugs can help to ease your symptoms until the results of behavioral and other therapies "kick in." It's also important to be compliant with medications while they are being prescribed so that you get the best possible result.

The bad news is that most of these medications may have one or more of the following side effects:

- dry mouth
- constipation
- abdominal pain
- nausea
- headaches
- insomnia
- anxiety and nervousness
- increased blood pressure
- blurred vision
- heartburn
- heart palpitations
- glaucoma
- decreased sweating
- drowsiness

There is another option to treat stress incontinence called **the impressa**. It is a disposable, tampon-like device. Each impressa is inserted inside the vagina and can be used for up to eight hours at a time. The first time you use it, you buy the sizing kit. There are three sizes and you start with the smallest and increase the size until it is comfortable. After you use the impressa for eight hours, you throw it away. Take a new one the next time one is necessary. This is a great option if you only have incontinence during specific activities such as working out or playing tennis or golf.

TECH TERMS

Anticholinergic drugs, used for urge incontinence, block the impulses between the nerves that control the bladder and the bladder muscle itself. The response of muscle to stimulation is chemically suppressed. These drugs stop or delay muscle spasms.

The good news is that most people taking these medications are unaffected or very mildly affected by the above conditions. Most patients who are affected do not stop taking the drug. Best of all, the side effects can be controlled by the size of the dosage. Dry mouth is the most common adverse effect. It is important to note that doctors have recently been warned about possible memory impairment in the elderly who take anticholinergic medications for an extended period of time.

There is a newer class of medication called beta-3 agonists. This medication, Mirabegron, causes the bladder to relax. People with high blood pressure need to be careful as the medication can increase blood pressure. Mirabegron does not cause possible memory impairment.

TECH TERMS

Sympathomimetic drugs, used for stress incontinence, tighten the muscles at the bladder neck. They cannot be taken with most drugs for Parkinson's disease or with drugs for high blood pressure. Beware! They may cause hypertensive reactions, headache, nausea, vomiting, and palpitations.[82] They have also not been cleared by the FDA for this use.

When a doctor prescribes a medication for you, be sure to ask the following questions:

- What can I expect this medication to do for me?
- How often will I have to take it?
- How is this medication taken—with food? On an empty stomach?
- What are the possible side effects?
- What side effects indicate that I should stop taking this medication immediately?
- Are there any restrictions involved? Can I drive? Drink alcoholic beverages? Should I avoid certain foods? Sunlight?
- Will this medication conflict with any other prescription medications I am currently taking?
- Will this medication conflict with any over-the-counter medications, vitamins, herbal, or alternative products I am currently taking?
- How long will I have to take it?

Consult the chart below for the most common medications prescribed today for urge incontinence.

DOS AND DON'TS

Before taking any medication for any condition, consult your physician first. A call to your pharmacist might also be a good idea. Never, ever self-prescribe medicine!

---

82   Choe JM. Pubovaginal Sling. eMedicine [Internet]. Section 6.

Drugs that treat urge incontinence

Antimuscarinics:
Darifenacin (Enablex)

Fesoterodine (Toviaz)

Oxybutynin (Ditropan, Ditropan XL)

Oxybutynin patch (Oxytrol)

Solifenacin (Vesicare)

Tolterodine (Detrol, Detrol LA)

Trospium (Sanctura)

Beta-3 agonists
Mirabegron (Myrbetriq)

Other medications for urge incontinence:
Dicyclomine (Bentyl)

Hyoscyamine (Levbid)

Imipramine (Tofranil)

Percutaneous Tibial Nerve Stimulation (PTNS)

When medications do not work, or the side effects are too much and you are not ready for surgery, percutaneous tibial nerve stimulation (PTNS) may be helpful. PTNS is an outpatient treatment option for patients with overactive bladder. It is unclear exactly why it has the results it does, but it does help many patients. This procedure involves inserting a small, acupuncture-like electrode on the inner side of the ankle. Once the electrode is placed, a pulsating signal sends messages to the bladder. A session lasts thirty minutes and is once a week for twelve consecutive weeks. Studies show that PTNS benefits approximately 60 percent of patients (similar to patient response to medication).[83] Other studies show that the effects last thirty months for daytime symptoms and eighteen

---

83 Gormley, E. A., Lightner, D. J., Faraday, M., & Vasavada, S. P. (2015). Diagnosis and treatment of overactive bladder (non-neurogenic) in adults: AUA/SUFU guideline amendment. *The Journal of urology*, 193(5), 1572-1580

months for nighttime symptoms.[84] One of the benefits of PTNS is that it is well-tolerated with very few side effects, if any. Unfortunately, patients with a pacemaker cannot get PTNS.

Just a few years ago, incontinence was a condition that no one discussed. Let's face it: it's really, really embarrassing. Today, however, incontinence is much more openly discussed, and ads for medications and adult diapers regularly appear in magazines and on television. It's about time.

Fortunately, in the race to garner the largest share of the consumer market, manufacturers of medications and other products to treat incontinence are constantly working to improve their products.

The Wrap-Up

- The first step toward bladder continence is behavioral bladder training which gradually increases the time between voiding episodes ("mind over bladder").
- Kegel exercises help strengthen your muscles and quiet unstable bladder contractions. Continuing to do them will lead to improvement in both urge and stress incontinence.
- Using cones and weights with Kegel exercises also helps strengthen pelvic muscles.
- Pessaries are mechanical devices that may be used to control incontinence and prolapse in lieu of surgery.
- Biofeedback therapy helps you to recognize how well you are controlling your pelvic muscles and bladder contractions and how your muscle strength is improving.
- Medication has been proven highly effective in controlling urge incontinence but less effective in controlling other forms of incontinence.
- PTNS is an excellent option for patients who prefer to avoid taking medication and are reluctant to opt for a more invasive procedure.

---

84 Del Río-Gonzalez, S., Aragon, I. M., Castillo, E., Milla-España, F., Galacho, A., Machuca, J., & Herrera-Imbroda, B. (2017). Percutaneous tibial nerve stimulation therapy for overactive bladder syndrome: clinical effectiveness, urodynamic, and durability evaluation. *Urology*, 108, 52-58.

11

Going Under the Knife
When It's Your Best Option

Chapter Highlights

- Surgery as an Option
- Selecting a Surgeon
- Surgeries for Stress Incontinence
- Surgeries for Urge Incontinence
- The Wrap-Up

For some of us, the path to continence is paved with Kegel exercises, bladder training, biofeedback machines, pills, cones, and/or pessaries. For others, however, the trip is a little more arduous, and surgery is a necessity. Take heart! There are many different surgical options available today for incontinence, and the overwhelming majority of them have a very high success rate, as you shall soon see. It's true that surgery is unpleasant, inconvenient, costly, and has its risks. And guidelines from the Agency for Health Care Policy and Research (AHCPR) state that conservative strategies should be stressed and that the first choice of a procedure for a patient should be the least invasive and least dangerous. But ladies, if surgery is the only way you'll be able to throw away those diapers forever and regain your freedom, it's an option you must consider. Read on to learn more about the different surgical options available today.

Surgery as an Option

Surgery for incontinence may be a medical necessity or it may be elective. This depends on each individual's unique situation, which should be discussed with a doctor. There are certain rare situations in which severe prolapse compromises one or both kidneys (so that surgery must be performed quickly), but this is the exception, not the rule. If the symptoms of incontinence don't bother you and don't hinder your lifestyle, there's no need to endure an operation unless you choose to. Some women would be satisfied if they only leaked a little and could get away with using pads or diapers, while others want to be completely dry.

Your doctor will evaluate your overall health and will investigate the specific cause of your incontinence. You must examine your personal symptoms and goals and then, after listening to the sound medical advice your doctor has to offer, make the decision that is best for you. There are many things to consider, and you may have to make a trade-off along the way. Keep the following in mind:

- All surgery has its risks, and the more complex the surgery, the greater the chance of complications.
- Simple surgeries generally have shorter recuperation periods but may have lower success rates.
- In some operations, the surgeon may make a small incision on the patient's abdomen (laparoscopic or robotic surgery) or may make a longer incision along the bikini line (abdominal surgery). Other operations may be performed through the vagina without requiring a visible cut (vaginal surgery).
- Maintaining a healthy weight is essential. Surgery is more difficult, runs an increased risk of complications, and has a lower success rate in people who are overweight.

Selecting a Surgeon

Of course, you want the best doctor on the planet to perform your surgery. How do you go about finding the best surgeon for you? First and foremost, it's a good idea to get a second (or even a third) opinion to ensure that the type of surgery suggested is the best course of action for you. Then you need to interview each prospective surgeon thoroughly. Take someone along with you who will listen attentively with you and take notes. Don't be intimidated by those impressive medical degrees on the wall. Ask a lot of questions. Remember that no question asked sincerely is stupid. The success of your surgery depends on the person performing it. Here is what you may want to ask:

- Where did you train and what is your specialty?
- Are you board certified in obstetrics and gynecology or urology?
- Did you take a registered fellowship in urogynecology?
- What is the best way to treat my problem?
- Are there any non-invasive alternatives to surgery?
- How many of these procedures have you performed?
- What is your success rate for the particular operation you will be performing on me?
- What, if any, are the potential risks involved?
- What are the chances that I will need surgery again after this procedure?
- Will this operation help my incontinence and by how much?
- What is done during this surgery?
- How long is my expected recovery time?
- What help will I need at home?
- Will I experience pain? If so, for how long? What will be suggested to reduce the pain?
- What is your hospital affiliation?
- What is the accreditation of the facility where you will perform my surgery?
- Who will administer anesthesia during my surgery?
- Can I meet the anesthesiologist before surgery to discuss issues, including what type of anesthesia will be offered?

Don't jump to have surgery immediately. This is a serious step you're considering here. Give yourself time to digest all the information you receive and to discuss it with family members and friends. If necessary, set up another appointment with the doctor to discuss your concerns, any remaining questions, and all the details of the operation.

Surgeries for Stress Incontinence

Surgeries for stress incontinence include:
- Bladder Neck Injections
- Sling Procedures
- Tension Free Transvaginal and Transobturator Tape
- Cystourethropexies

Bladder Neck Injections

This procedure involves the injection of synthetic bulking agents (generally tiny silicone particles or other types of small particles) into the wall of the uppermost part of the urethra (bladder neck). This is done to improve the urethra's ability to resist opening and to strengthen it so that urine can't leak out. This minimally invasive "surgery" is usually performed in a doctor's office on women with a weakened urethral sphincter condition (intrinsic sphincter deficiency—ISD). Bladder neck injection is contraindicated in the case of a urinary tract infection or with untreated overactive bladder/urge incontinence.

Currently available agents for periurethral bladder neck injections include:
- carbon-coated zirconium oxide beads suspended in a water-based gel (Durasphere).
- cross-linked polydimethylsiloxane (Macroplastique) or polydimethylsiloxane (Urolastic).
- calcium hydroxyapatite suspended in a water and glycerine gel (Coaptite).

The advantages of a bladder neck injection are:
- It is minimally invasive.
- It is useful for women who want to avoid open surgery.
- It is valuable for women with ISD and in women with ISD who use a pessary.
- It can be used to correct residual mild stress incontinence after a surgical procedure.
- Complication rates are low.

Disadvantages are:

- It has a low long-term cure rate.
- The injections may have to be repeated several times.

Sling Procedures

All types of stress incontinence may be corrected with sling surgery. In a sling procedure, a sling (like a hammock) is passed under the urethra and attached to the connective tissue of the abdominal wall. The sling moves with any increase of abdominal pressure so that during a cough, for example, the sling itself moves up, stabilizing the urethra, increasing its pressure, and preventing leakage.

A number of different materials can be used by surgeons to construct slings:

- Tissues from the patient's body can be harvested at the time of surgery (from connective tissue from the abdominal wall or thigh). This is called a pubovaginal, or fascial sling, and is usually reserved for patients for whom other surgeries for stress incontinence have failed.
- The use of synthetic materials, such as polypropylene, allows for a shorter operating time and results in long-term outcomes similar to those of more invasive procedures. These materials may, however, cause vaginal and urethral tissue erosion. Their long-term cure rate is high, varying from 75 to 85 percent.[85]

Although complications from sling surgery are rare, patients should be counseled about the potential risks of these procedures, including: bleeding, infection, injury to the bladder, the bowel, the urethra, urethral obstruction (from a sling that overly restricts or narrows the urethra), new onset or worsening of urge incontinence, and urinary retention (in 2 to 9 percent of patients).[86] Although urinary retention is generally temporary, it may last for as long as a month or more. Patients, therefore, should also be made aware that this surgery may require post-operative self-catheterization. A second operation to improve urinary retention is usually not necessary.

---

85   Op cit. Choe JM. Section 7.
86   Ibid. Section 6.

Tension Free Transvaginal and Transobturator Tape

Tension Free Vaginal Tape (TVT) is a polypropylene mesh tape that is used to recreate support under the urethra. The TVT is a minimally invasive and simple outpatient surgical option that can usually be completed in less than an hour under general anesthesia. A small incision is made in the vagina and the tape is placed around the mid-urethra in a U shape. It exits through two small incisions in the lower abdomen just above the pubic bone. It is secured in place by friction and heals, over time, by scarring. This sling supports the middle of the urethra and allows it to keep its "seal" when needed, without unnecessary tension. It also helps prevent the downward trend of the urethra that occurs with stress.

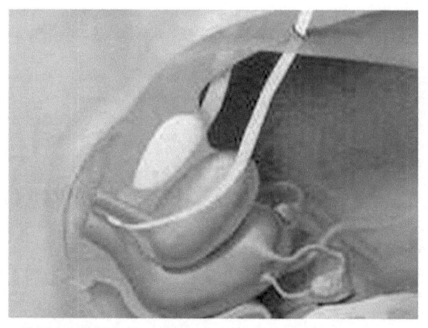

The Gynecare TVT in Place. Reproduced with permission. © ETHICON, INC.

The transobturator tape (TOT), another type of sling procedure, is very similar to the TVT. Both procedures elevate and support the urethra in times of increased abdominal stress by placing the tape around the mid-urethra. The difference is that the tape exits from a different place for the TVT (through the skin above the pubic bone) and for the TOT (through the skin on the inside of the thighs). Cure rates for the TVT and TOT are excellent.

There is also a single incision sling (mini-sling) that appears to be effective, however, more long-term data is currently needed to evaluate its efficacy. This procedure is very similar to the TOT sling, but eliminates the need for exit incisions.

Some of the complications of sling procedures include: bladder perforation injury to blood vessels and bowel, difficulty urinating, and erosion of the vagina. Complications are treatable as long as they are recognized quickly. Some patients go home with a Foley catheter for a few days to drain the urine.

Cystourethropexies

Named for the surgeons who perfected them, the Burch and Marshall-Marchetti-Krantz operations are performed in the lower abdomen with a single incision, or with multiple small incisions (robotic surgery). The object of the surgery is to correct the improper position of the bladder neck resulting from stress. The surgeon ties several sutures in the connective tissue alongside the urethra to support it and the vagina. The bladder neck is repositioned into an anatomically normal position so that it remains closed during periods of increased physical activity. As a result, urinary incontinence is dramatically reduced. Most studies agree that these procedures have an excellent long-term cure rate. It is advantageous that they may be performed laparoscopically or robotically. This procedure is perfect for women with a good, intact internal urethral sphincter. However, because it is more invasive than TVT, TVT is more commonly performed.

Be aware that this surgery does have some rare complications:
- Difficulty urinating, which may require catheterization
- Painful urination
- Infection
- Blood loss
- Damage to the bladder

TECH TERMS

Laparoscopy/Robotic Surgery is a procedure in which the surgeon uses a small video camera and a few specialized instruments to perform surgery with minimal tissue injury. The camera and instruments are inserted through small skin incisions that allow the surgeon to explore the entire area and perform the required surgery without having to make large incisions.

BELIEVE IT OR NOT

With all of my incontinence problems I have, fortunately, never had to consider surgery. My trials and tribulations were plentiful, but conventional treatments worked for me. I kept a diary, I did bladder training, I did (and still do) Kegels, I took medication, I used cones, I plugged in to a variety of biofeedback machines, and I did hours of physical therapy to become cured.

But not all of us are so lucky. And some of us are just downright impatient or want a quick fix without having to do any work. The latter was the case of Ms. X.

My friend, Terry, is an O.R. nurse at a major neighborhood hospital. She comes home with stories that make you wonder about people and where their heads are. On the evening in question, Terry had a long conversation with Ms. X as she lied there on the operating table. It seems that Ms. X was a very busy person, such a busy person that she had no time for the less invasive treatments for dealing with uterine prolapse. She wanted no part of bladder diaries, medication, Kegels, and certainly no part of vaginal cones. And there was no way she would condescend to stick a biofeedback probe into her vagina.

Ms. X opted for surgery so that she could get immediate results effortlessly. And she chose an epidural (spinal block) as her means of anesthesia so that she could be awake and entertained during the operation. And so she chatted incessantly with my friend, Terry, telling her all the gory details of her latest love adventure.

Midway through the procedure, the conversation was abruptly interrupted when Terry heard a funny sound emanating from under the sterile surgical sheets draped around Ms. X's midsection. Both Terry and the surgeon couldn't believe it when Ms. X whipped out her cellphone and started talking to her stockbroker. Apparently, her stocks were taking a nosedive. Fortunately for Ms. X, no one else in the operating room was even remotely affected by the bad news.

Surgeries for Urge Incontinence

Surgeries for urge incontinence include:

- Botulinum Toxin A Bladder Injections (Botox Injections)
- Sacral Nerve Neuromodulation
- Augmentation Cytoplasty
- Urinary Diversion

Botulinum Toxin A Bladder Injections (Botox Injections)

The bladder acts like a balloon: as urine is produced and enters the bladder, the bladder wall needs to expand. As the bladder fills, you start to get the urge to go to the bathroom. Once you have decided to empty your bladder, the bladder contracts and you urinate. If you have overactive bladder, you cannot control when the bladder decides to contract and you may have accidents. For example, patients with spinal cord damage experience a disruption between the signals in the spinal cord and bladder and, as a result, frequently have overactive bladder. When medications for overactive bladder do not work or cannot be tolerated, another treatment option is Botulinum Toxin A (Botox Injections).

Botox can be injected into the bladder muscle, causing it to relax. As a result, urgency, frequency, and incontinence are reduced. The effects of Botox generally last from three to nine months and, in some cases, even longer. The procedure can be performed in a doctor's office. First, a local anesthetic is administered.

Then, a cystoscope is inserted and a small needle is used to inject the Botox. After the treatment, the patient can go home. Antibiotics may be prescribed before and/or after the procedure. It may take up to two weeks for the Botox to work.

Pregnant patients, patients with a urinary tract infection, and those with a history of myasthenia gravis or Eaton-Lambert syndrome should not get Botox. There are some risks, which include: urinary tract infection, allergic reaction, and temporary inability to empty your bladder. Overall, Botox is extremely effective and there is a 60 to 90 percent chance of significant improvement in symptoms.[87]

Sacral Nerve Neuromodulation

The sacral nerve runs from the lower spinal cord to the bladder and is responsible for stimulating the muscles and organs involved in bladder control and pelvic floor contractions. Sacral nerve neuromodulation (**Medtronic InterStim System**) provides sacral nerve stimulation and treats severe urinary urge incontinence or urinary retention, as well as fecal incontinence, in patients who have failed to respond to, or could not tolerate, more conservative, non-invasive treatments.

Prior to the implantation of the **InterStim** therapy system, a test stimulation procedure is done to assess how well the nerves function. This is a simple outpatient procedure that is performed under local anesthesia. The device is placed under the skin in the patient's lower back. The electrodes attached to it exit the patient's body and are attached to an external pacemaker that the patient can wear like a pager or beeper. The system is worn for up to two week, and the patient must keep a diary in which she records her symptoms. If improvement is noted, the patient is a good candidate for surgical implantation of the permanent electrode.

If the patient opts for surgery, the **InterStim** system is permanently placed in the operating room during a second procedure. A small, implantable device (that resembles a pacemaker) sends mild electrical impulses to the sacral nerve, located in the lower back above the tailbone. This **InterStim** device is implanted under the skin in the patient's abdomen. A wire from the device is attached to the sacral nerve. Painless electrical pulses travel through this wire to the sacral nerve

---

87   https://www.yourpelvicfloor.org/

in an effort to improve or eliminate bladder control symptoms that may lead to overflow incontinence. The impulses decrease the bladder muscle's sensitivity and, therefore, decrease bladder contractions and the urge incontinence that results from these contractions. A special program allows the doctor to customize and adjust settings and to check the information being given by the neurostimulator. A portable patient programmer has an on-off switch for the neurostimulator and allows the patient to check the status of the battery and to adjust the stimulation level within the levels set by the doctor.

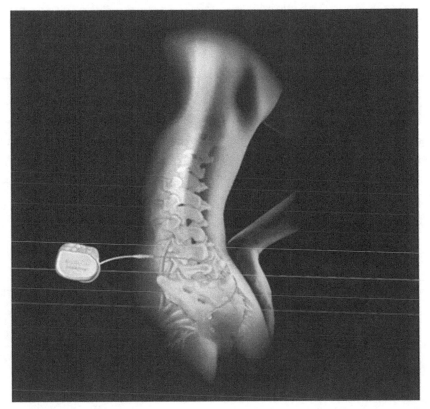

The InterStim System in Place. Reprinted with permission. Courtesy of Medtronic, Inc.

The advantages of sacral nerve stimulation are:
- It is safe.
- It is reversible. The device can be removed.

- It does not preclude use of another procedure for treating urinary incontinence.

Q&A

How long does the* InterStim *battery last, and will it interfere with other electronic devices?

The **InterStim** battery life is anywhere from five to nine years, with seven to nine years as the average. Rechargeable batteries are being developed. The stimulator is safe to use around the house and does not interfere with home appliances. Possible complications include infection and tissue damage.

Augmentation Cystoplasty

Augmentation cystoplasty is a major operation performed for severe urge incontinence only when all other available procedures and treatments have proven ineffective. When the bladder is no longer able to store urine, due to muscle damage from overfilling or due to uncontrollable contractions, this procedure may help the patient by increasing the capacity of her bladder (the amount of urine her bladder can hold prior to urination) and by preventing it from contracting involuntarily. This surgery involves taking a piece of the patient's intestine and using it to enlarge and reconstruct the bladder. The most common complications associated with this surgery are:

- Difficulty urinating (retention).
- Recurrent urinary incontinence (requiring self-catheterization).
- Bowel obstruction or diarrhea.
- Bleeding.
- Infection.

Urinary Diversion

When the bladder and/or urethra are damaged beyond repair and no longer serve a useful function, urinary diversion surgery is the only option available.

In one type of diversion surgery, a piece of intestine is used to construct a urinary reservoir that serves as a new bladder that collects urine. Another piece of intestine may be shaped to function as the urethra would. It remains attached to the existing urethra or it exits the body through the abdomen. The patient either voids through the new urethra or by means of intermittent self-catheterization.

This operation can lead to complications, such as damage to bowel, bladder, and surrounding tissues and additional surgery may become necessary.

The Wrap-Up

- Surgery is a viable option in the treatment of stress and urge incontinence. Surgery may be recommended only after non-invasive options have been tried.

- Select a surgeon only after doing considerable research and after asking many questions.

- Bladder neck injections use synthetic bulking agents to strengthen the urethral wall in order to prevent urine leakage. These injections are used to treat stress incontinence, especially ISD (intrinsic sphincter deficiency).

- Sling procedures (TVT, TOT, or pubovaginal sling) are used to treat stress incontinence. A sling, using either the patient's own tissue or synthetic materials, lifts and supports the urethra and bladder neck, especially during times of physical stress. These procedures may be performed vaginally, abdominally, or laparoscopically.

- Botulinum Toxin A Bladder Injections or Botox injections into the bladder muscle can be done in a doctor's office and are a great option for patients who cannot tolerate medications.

- Cystourethropexies are bladder neck suspension procedures used to treat stress incontinence. They support the urethra without increasing its inside pressure.

- Sacral nerve stimulation requires the implantation of a device that electrically stimulates the sacral nerve which, in turn, is responsible for stimulating muscles and organs involved in bladder control and pelvic floor contractions. This procedure is performed on patients with severe urge incontinence who do not respond to or cannot tolerate more conservative treatments.

- Augmentation cystoplasty is used to treat severe urge incontinence when other treatments have proven unsuccessful. This surgery reconstructs the bladder with a section of bowel.
- Urinary diversion is used when the bladder or urethra is damaged beyond repair and no other treatment options are available.

Extraordinary People/ Extraordinary Situations

Chapter Highlights

- Pregnant Women
- Menopausal Women
- Seniors
- Women with Interstitial Cystitis
- Women with Injuries and Birth Defects
- Women with Diabetes
- Women with Multiple Sclerosis
- Stroke Victims
- Women with Parkinson's Disease
- Women with Alzheimer's and Dementia
- The Wrap-Up

In our own special way, each and every one of us is an extraordinary person. Think about it! Along life's paths we've all found ourselves in some very extraordinary situations. I know I have. But when it comes to bladder control and bladder function, there are those among us who are faced with greater difficulties and who require more patience, more help, and more understanding. Look around and you will notice that you know someone like that. I do. I'm thinking of Grandma Rose, who spent her last years in a nursing home, where the air was permeated with the acrid stench of dried urine. Then there's my twenty-three-year-old second cousin, who, due to a birth defect, is still in diapers and requires dialysis until a new kidney can be found. I also think about my friend's five-year-old, who was born with a rare genetic disease and will need extensive physical therapy in the future to become continent; my beautiful, talented aunt with Alzheimer's, who doesn't remember to use the bathroom; and my cousin's wife with multiple sclerosis who, despite taking every medication known to mankind to stave off the effects of her debilitating disease, must cope with problems of poor bladder control.

I could go on and on, but you get the picture. This final chapter is for and about those with special needs, those for whom incontinence presents a very difficult challenge.

Pregnant Women

Were you ever pregnant? Do you remember what it felt like? Of course it was an exhilarating experience, but who could ever forget the discomforts? Pregnancy makes your bladder work overtime. Right from the outset, it makes your kidneys produce more urine, increasing your urge to urinate more frequently. Increased pressure on your bladder as your uterus enlarges, brought about by that constantly growing bundle of joy you are carrying, has the same result. Your hormones are in a state of flux, and the tissues in your pelvis relax and become more flexible, which may cause you to leak. If you're pregnant, you may feel that you can't completely empty your bladder, and you'll make many uncomfortable trips to the bathroom.

DOS AND DON'TS

Do try to keep your weight under control during pregnancy to avoid excess pressure on your bladder. Maintaining a healthy weight before pregnancy will lessen your chances of bladder and uterine prolapse and the resulting stress incontinence that may accompany it. One word of caution, however: don't diet during your pregnancy in an attempt to save your bladder. A healthy weight gain (depending, of course, upon your starting weight and your build) is anywhere between twenty-four and thirty-six pounds.

By the third trimester of pregnancy, during the day you may be urinating every time you turn around, and during the night you may find yourself sitting on the potty two to three times, when you'd much rather be sleeping. You may have an accident or two during your pregnancy. You may suffer from urge incontinence, stress incontinence, or a combination of the two, and your problems might become more severe with each successive pregnancy. Hopefully, all of these symptoms will disappear after the fact. But, of course, first you have to contend with childbirth.

All the changes your body undergoes weaken your natural defenses and leave you more susceptible than ever to urinary tract infections. Although rare, urinary retention is a problem that may sometimes lead to overflow incontinence. This condition may occur if the growing uterus presses the urethra against the pubic bone, blocking the flow of urine.

BELIEVE IT OR NOT

I was young and stupid and ecstatically pregnant for the very first time. My doctor was a traditional, conservative man and wasn't a big fan of sharing medical information with his patients. So he never told me, throughout my entire pregnancy, that my little son inside was an obstinate, contrary creature who was destined to present as a breech delivery—feet first. He also never revealed the benefits of Kegel exercises to prevent or minimize any damage that might occur from childbirth.

I had an easy pregnancy and felt fine, so I continued to work as a teacher. Laws had just been passed that prohibited the Board of Education from making a pregnant teacher take a leave of absence in her seventh month, and I was delighted to take advantage of the new rules.

One day in my third trimester, I was teaching a reading lesson, when I heard a disturbance at the back of the room. I stopped my lesson and decided to take a look. As I had expected, there was Peter Cardone drawing psychedelic creatures on his recently cleaned and scrubbed desk. With a smile on my face, I went to the rear closet to hand him a sponge and some gritty cleanser. On my way back to the front, my little boy gave me such a violent kick with his tiny left foot that I fell down onto my left knee and felt a trickle of urine run down my right leg. The students gasped as I stopped breathing for a moment. I was saved from major embarrassment by my opaque black tights, which hid the stream going down my leg. From that day on, I wore pads, just in case.

Childbirth is not without its bladder risks. Stretching and tearing of pelvic tissues occurs in pregnancy from the weight of the baby, the placenta, and the amniotic fluid. A vaginal delivery will stretch and may permanently damage the pelvic muscles and support structures, causing pelvic organ prolapse. The pudendal nerve, which controls the muscles of the pelvic floor, may also sustain enough damage to cause prolapse and incontinence after childbirth. The episiotomy, which may be performed to prevent tears to the pelvic muscles, may also injure the same muscles it is trying to protect. On the other hand, if no episiotomy is done, the resulting tears can injure the pelvic nerves, muscles, and connective tissues, which may contribute to future prolapse and incontinence. There really is no place for a routine episiotomy as part of any twenty-first-century birthing plan. This cut may be performed by a doctor on a case-by-case basis in order to maximize the overall health of the mother and baby. Don't think that a caesarean section will necessarily protect your pelvic floor from damage either. Damage to nerves, muscles, and connective tissues may occur during the surgery.

TECH TERMS

An **episiotomy** is the cut made in the lower portion of the pelvic muscles during childbirth to prevent these muscles from tearing irregularly, possibly causing damage.

Menopausal Women

In my humble opinion, whoever said that menopause was a wonderful, liberating time for women must have had a totally different experience than I did. I don't know about the rest of you out there in the over-fifty crowd, but losing my estrogen was about as bad as losing my best friend. Honestly, give me back my period with all its inconveniences! Enduring menstruation beats feeling like a dried-up prune! When our estrogen levels drop dramatically, our estrogen-sensitive pelvic muscles, nerves, connective tissue, and skin lose their strength and begin to atrophy as the collagen in them weakens. Surface skin becomes thinner and less lubricated. Our bladder, our bowel, and our uterus lose support, and prolapse may occur. That's when, in addition to night sweats, sleeplessness, mood swings, hot flashes, and painful intercourse, we may also experience urgency, frequency, dysuria (difficulty in urination), and urinary incontinence. Not fun.

As if menopause wasn't bad enough, a condition called atrophic vaginitis may occur when estrogen levels are low and the levels of bacteria, and their delicate balance within the vagina, change. The vaginal walls damage more easily and become thin and inflamed; you itch, and you may feel just plain sore. Some women experience atrophic vaginitis after childbirth or while breastfeeding, when estrogen levels are low. Should your urethra become irritated as a result of this condition, you'll probably feel the need to urinate more frequently.

TECH TERMS

Atrophic vaginitis is a condition in which the vagina becomes inflamed due to tissues that shrink and become thin as a result of decreased lubrication of the vaginal walls. This condition is caused by the lack of estrogen normally associated with menopause.

Seniors

Have you looked in the mirror lately and wept? Well, I have. I look at a face that I find difficult to recognize. My once beautiful, long, dark hair looks and feels limp and dried out despite the gobs of conditioner I treat it to on a daily basis. My skin looks like it was injected with cottage cheese, and it sags despite the hours and hours of cardio and weight training I do each week. Keeping all that in mind, there must be earth-shattering internal changes as well.

Q&A

So what happens to our bladder as we age?

Our bladder sensation changes and we don't feel the need to urinate until our bladder is almost full. For those of us with an overactive bladder, that means that we get less warning before we really have to go. And that could lead to accidents.

Our greatest amount of urine is produced at night, because our kidneys work more efficiently and make urine faster when we are lying down and inactive. Seniors suffering from nocturia, who have to get up several times during the night to use the bathroom, risk falling and hurting themselves as they hurry to void. A commode in the bedroom, in this case, is not a bad idea. You could always disguise it as a planter during the daytime! Seriously, in the dark, it may save you from slipping and falling on your "puddle" on your way to the bathroom.

Our bladder capacity decreases because our muscles shrink and can't hold as much urine as they used to. And so we urinate more frequently.

Our urinary stream strength diminishes.

Women with Interstitial Cystitis

Interstitial cystitis (IC) is not your common, everyday variety of bladder infection, because it is not caused by bacteria. It is a chronic, severe, debilitating inflammatory syndrome of the bladder that causes frequent, urgent, painful urination and pelvic discomfort in women. It is often misdiagnosed. A proper diagnosis requires that a doctor take urine cultures and tests and conduct specific bladder tests, such as cystoscopy (looking inside the bladder). The individuals who suffer from interstitial cystitis have bladders that are inflamed, easily irritated, scarred, and tender, and their bladders don't store urine well. They feel discomfort, pressure, tenderness, or intense pain in their bladder and pelvic area. In other words, their bladders are hypersensitive and they experience urgency and/or frequency as their bladders fill.

Signs of interstitial cystitis are:

- An urgent need to urinate.
- Urinary frequency where only a small amount of urine is voided.
- Pain in the lower abdomen and/or in the area between the vagina and the anus.
- Pain before, during, or after sexual intercourse.
- Chronic pelvic pain.

According to the National Institute of Health (NIH), interstitial cystitis affects between three and eight million women in the United States.[88] Its cause is currently unknown, although many theories exist as to why it occurs:

- Some believe that the bladder wall allows certain harmful bacteria to penetrate it. The bladder wall is generally lined with, and protected

---

88   www.ichelp.org/about-ic/what-is-interstitial-cystitis/4-to-12-million-may-have-ic.

by, a layer of protein called glycosaminoglycan (GAG) that shields the bladder from the invasion of toxins and chemicals. Patients with IC are believed to have a reduced or broken-down protective GAG layer.

- Another theory is that it is a negative autoimmune response, provoked by a bladder infection, wherein healthy cells are attacked.
- It is believed that pelvic floor muscle spasms may be to blame.
- Another premise is that there is an increased number of mast cells in the bladder wall. Mast cells are found in many different tissues. They play an important role in allergic reactions by defending our bodies against invading organisms, especially in wound healing. The mast cells secrete chemicals that cause pain.
- Certain abnormalities in the bladder wall are, perhaps, to blame.
- Interstitial cystitis may be genetic.

IC sufferers may also experience: asthma, endometriosis, food allergies, hay fever, incontinence, irritable bowel syndrome, fibromyalgia, lupus, migraine headaches, rheumatoid arthritis, and sinusitis. What is the connection between these conditions and IC? No one seems to know.[89]

If you believe that you suffer from interstitial cystitis, you need to visit your doctor, who will probably perform a cystoscopy (see chapter 4) to rule out a urinary tract infection, kidney stones, bladder cancer, sexually transmitted diseases, endometriosis, vaginal infection, or another condition that may just be masquerading as IC. If, however, IC is found, treatments are available.

Treatment for interstitial cystitis includes non-invasive techniques such as:

- Diet modification. IC symptoms may be reduced by avoiding caffeine in beverages and in chocolate, carbonated drinks, all citrus products, foods containing a high concentration of vitamin C, spicy and acidic foods, pickled foods, artificial sweeteners, and alcohol.
- Stress-reduction exercises.
- Pelvic floor relaxation exercises.
- Biofeedback.

---

89 www.mayoclinc.com. Interstitial cystitis. Treatment.

- Bladder retraining once pain has been controlled.
- Medications including:
  - Antidepressants to relieve pain: amitriptyline or imipramine, as well as several others.
  - Antihistamines for their sedative and anxiety-reducing effects: hydroxyzine pamoate, hydroxyzine hydrochloride and cromolyn sodium.
  - Pentodan polysulfate sodium, which eases the pain and discomfort of IC.
  - Muscle relaxants and analgesics to relieve chronic symptoms.
  - Antispasmodics, anticholinergics, H2 blockers, urinary alkalizing agents, adrenergic blockers, and leukotriene inhibitors.
- Bladder instillation, which is a type of bladder wash or bath. A catheter is used to fill the bladder with liquid medicine for anywhere from a few seconds to fifteen minutes before being emptied. Treatments are given every one to two weeks for six to eight weeks, can be repeated as often as necessary, and are frequently performed under sedation.
- Transcutaneous electrical nerve stimulation (TENS), which delivers mild electric pulses that block pain signals to the bladder. This technique helps relieve pain and urinary frequency in some IC sufferers.
- Sacral nerve modulation, which is also being studied as another way to relieve IC symptoms. (See chapter 11).
- An injection of Botulin (Botulism Toxin), which greatly reduces the pain of IC in some IC sufferers.

Surgery is only recommended to treat interstitial cystitis as a last resort because it is invasive and irreversible. There is also the possibility that some patients may find that their symptoms do not improve and may even become worse. Surgical options, which have minimal effectiveness, include:

- Bladder augmentation: The damaged portion of the patient's bladder is replaced with a piece of intestine. This surgery often necessitates the use of a catheter several times a day (See chapter 11).

- Fulguration: Instruments are inserted through the urethra to cauterize ulcers that may be present.
- Resection: Instruments are inserted through the urethra to remove ulcers.[90]

DOS AND DON'TS

For help coping with interstitial cystitis, contact the Interstitial Cystitis Association on the internet at www.ichelp.org or call 703-442-2070

Women with Injuries and Birth Defects

Women with birth defects (such as spina bifida), or those with spinal cord injuries and neurologic impairment (paraplegics and quadriplegics), suffer from reflex incontinence as a result of damage to the central nervous system. The brain can no longer receive messages from the bladder, so control is lost, and continual incontinence, urinary retention, or incontinence after voiding occurs.

With reflex incontinence, a woman does not sense that she must urinate and doesn't feel the urge to void when the bladder contracts involuntarily. The bladder will empty itself unpredictably when it is full or in response to external stimuli such as cold air. Reflex incontinence can be managed by scheduled voiding, intermittent catheterization, or augmentation cystoplasty (see chapter 11). Proper treatment for reflex incontinence is needed to prevent kidney disease.

Women with Diabetes

Diabetes can adversely affect the bladder.

- If diabetes is not properly monitored and controlled with diet and/or medication, the blood sugar level may skyrocket, causing great thirst. The more you drink, the more you urinate. So urinary frequency can become a problem for those who suffer from diabetes.

---

90   www.mayoclinic.com. Multiple sclerosis. Overview. Signs and symptoms.

TECH TERMS

Myelin is a fatty protein that encases nerves. The myelin sheath is responsible for the proper transmission of nerve impulses.

- The myelin sheath that encases the nerves that go to the bladder becomes damaged. The ensuing nerve damage causes communication problems between the brain and the bladder, and the bladder and the sphincter cease to function normally. This condition is known as **diabetic cystopathy.**

The first indication of diabetes is reduced bladder sensations: the patient no longer feels the urge to urinate. This causes the bladder to distend (become bigger and bigger) until discomfort sets in and the urge to void presents itself. As a result, urination will be less frequent. As the bladder stretches and the muscles weaken, however, voiding becomes increasingly difficult. The patient may be totally unaware that a problem exists due to impaired bladder sensations.

If the condition is ignored, urine builds up in the bladder, leading to recurring infections, difficulty in urinating, overflow incontinence, and, eventually, possible kidney failure. With proper medical care and good, tight sugar control, diabetes should not present any major bladder problems. If, however, diabetic cystopathy is already an issue, it is usually irreversible and will require special treatment. Scheduled voiding is one way to manage the problem. Intermittent self-catheterization will be necessary if the bladder is irreparably damaged.

Women with Multiple Sclerosis

Multiple sclerosis is a chronic, debilitating, degenerative disease of the nervous system that affects more than one million people in the United States and is two to three times more common in women than in men.[91] First symptoms generally appear between the ages of twenty and forty. In people with multiple sclerosis,

---

91   https://www.healthline.com/health/multiple-sclerosis/facts-statistics-infographic#1.

the immune system mistakenly attacks and destroys the cells that produce the myelin sheath, the fatty protein that encases and protects nerve fibers.

At first, the myelin sheath becomes inflamed and swollen and detaches from the nerve fibers. In more severe cases, the myelin may be destroyed. Sclerosed (hardened) scar tissue forms over the nerve fibers, preventing nerve impulses from traveling to and from the brain in damaged areas, and causing many different kinds of neurologic symptoms. Eventually, this process leads to nerve degeneration, which causes the disabilities encountered by patients with multiple sclerosis: numbness or weakness in limbs, loss of vision, double or blurred vision, tingling or pain in numb areas, tremors, lack of coordination, fatigue, dizziness, slurred speech, and paralysis.[92]

Multiple sclerosis is characterized by an unpredictable, fluctuating loss of muscle strength and coordination. Bladder and bowel problems are common, due to the interruption and interference of nerve impulses between the brain and the bladder or colon. The loss of bladder or bowel control may be temporary or persistent, improving or becoming worse as the patient's symptoms ebb and flow.

The most common bladder problems experienced by women with multiple sclerosis are: urinary frequency, urgency, urge incontinence (generally caused by involuntary bladder contractions), urinary retention (incomplete bladder emptying that occurs when the sphincter doesn't open properly during a bladder contraction and urine isn't voided), nocturia (frequent night voiding), reflex incontinence, and bladder infection.

Bladder problems that result from multiple sclerosis are initially treated with the least invasive methods possible: Kegel exercises, medications, behavior modification, bladder training, and intermittent self-catheterization. Surgery is reserved for only the more advanced cases, when conservative methods of treating incontinence have failed.

Stroke Victims

After a stroke, many victims initially experience urinary frequency, urgency, and urge incontinence caused by involuntary bladder contractions. Some sufferers

---

92   NAFC. Quality Care. 20(1).

can't urinate at all. Urinary retention may also be an issue and may lead to overflow incontinence (see chapter 7). Reflex incontinence may also pose a problem. The good news is that most of these victims can expect an eventual recovery (either partial, or even full, in certain cases). The bad news is that this may take a bit of time and patience and can be a frustrating and depressing experience.

Women with Parkinson's Disease

Parkinson's disease is a slowly progressing, degenerative neurologic disease of the nervous system characterized by tremors, rigidity, a shuffling gait, and bladder problems. Stiff muscles may make it difficult for the patient to get to the bathroom in time, thus causing accidents. Weak nerves and sphincter muscles that control urination and bowel movements lead to urinary and fecal incontinence. Many patients with Parkinson's disease have urinary tract infections; urge incontinence, caused by involuntary bladder contractions that cause the patient to urinate without control; and reflex incontinence. Fortunately, there are some newer medications that can help control the symptoms of Parkinson's disease for quite a while.

Women with Alzheimer's Disease and Dementia

As they age, some women develop Alzheimer's disease or dementia (senility). Alzheimer's disease is a neurologic condition in which memory, speech, muscles, and the intellect variably and progressively deteriorate and worsen until the patient can no longer take care of her personal needs. Alzheimer's is characterized by dementia or gradual mental deterioration to the point where the patient loses her memory, her language and problem-solving skills, her ability to learn, her judgment, and her ability to perform daily activities. Patients who suffer from dementia do not necessarily have Alzheimer's.

In the early stages of both disorders, incontinence is not a problem unless some other condition is involved. As the disorders reach a more advanced stage, however, reflex incontinence occurs because the brain can no longer handle urinary control, causing the patient to urinate without warning. Due to memory loss and the loss of other cognitive processes, the patient may forget where it is appropriate to urinate and may void where she shouldn't. Scheduled voiding by a trained caregiver is an option to consider. If that fails, absorbent pads may become a necessity.

The Wrap-Up

- Pregnancy increases the urge to urinate as the enlarging uterus presses against the bladder.
- Lack of estrogen can cause the pelvic tissues to weaken and function poorly, which may result in prolapse and incontinence.
- As we age, our bladder sensations change, we produce more urine at night and have to get up more frequently, our bladder capacity decreases, and our urinary stream may be less forceful.
- Interstitial cystitis is a debilitating inflammatory condition in which the bladder is hypersensitive. It is not caused by bacteria and, to date, has no known cause.
- Women with spinal injuries, birth defects such as spina bifida, and neurologic impairment may suffer from reflex incontinence, where they do not sense the need or feel the urge to urinate.
- Women with diabetes can control any resultant bladder problem early on through proper medical and dietary management of the disease.
- Women with multiple sclerosis may suffer urinary and/or bowel incontinence as nerve impulses between the bladder and the brain are interrupted and their muscles lose their strength and coordination.
- Stroke victims may temporarily lose bladder control, which can be regained as the body heals.
- Women with Parkinson's disease have leakage accidents as a result of their loss of mobility due to stiff muscles.
- Women with Alzheimer's disease and dementia become incontinent as the disease advances because the brain loses its ability to control the bladder.

Afterword

The Ultimate Wrap-Up

At this point, we hope you're convinced that continence is a goal you can successfully attain or, at the very least, maximize for your particular situation with the help of a trained, understanding, compassionate medical practitioner. We hope we've given you the proper information to help you choose such a physician. Freedom and control are within your reach if you are proactive about your bladder health and are willing to take the necessary steps to deal with a problem that is treatable.

By now you've spent a considerable amount of time learning the detailed workings of the urinary tract: how your kidneys, your ureters, your bladder, your urethra, your sphincter muscles, your pelvic floor muscles, your spinal cord, and your brain are responsible for your continence or lack thereof.

We've presented you with the common risk factors for incontinence:

- age
- gender
- pelvic muscle weakness
- pregnancy
- childbirth
- menopause
- fluid intake
- constipation
- smoking

- obesity
- caffeine intake
- certain food products
- high impact physical activities
- urinary tract infections
- illness

These factors all affect the proper functioning of your bladder.

In addition, problems with the pelvic organs themselves (such as fibroids), pelvic organ prolapse, and the use of certain prescription drugs can also cause bladder problems. You may be able to recognize some of your symptoms. Share these with your doctor so that you can make continence a reality and not just a dream.

After reading this book and really hearing our message, you may be able to better listen to your body, feel how it works, and then make an educated decision about how you want to proceed. Don't be afraid to monitor your habits. Take precautions to prevent bladder infections.

If you feel there's still a problem, don't be shy or embarrassed. You're not alone, and there are kind, understanding professionals eager to help you. Seek out a referral to a physician familiar with the area of female urinary incontinence—either a urogynecologist or urologist—and make sure that you get a full work-up. You won't be sorry you did.

Make sure you understand the different types of incontinence:

- Stress incontinence is generally caused by weakness of the pelvic muscles (including the urethral sphincter and its nerves) or the connective tissues surrounding and supporting these muscles. Leakage of urine in these cases results when there is increased abdominal pressure due to coughing, jumping, or laughing or when the urethral sphincter simply cannot close properly. Non-invasive exercise programs can help the majority of women who suffer from this type of incontinence.
- Urge incontinence, caused by muscle spasms in the bladder wall itself, triggers the frequent, immediate need to void, often accompanied by

leakage. Some non-invasive treatments that we have mentioned include: behavioral therapy, physical therapy, and medications.

- Overflow incontinence is caused by a bladder that does not empty sufficiently during urination.
- Functional incontinence is usually found in older people. They may otherwise have good bladder control but, because of physical disabilities, are unable to use available toilet facilities.
- Reflex incontinence, caused by damaged nerves resulting from a neurological disorder, occurs in those who are unaware of the need to urinate.
- Fecal incontinence is the inability to voluntarily control bowel movements; to discriminate between solid, liquid, and gas; and to put off defecation until a socially convenient time. Non-invasive treatments include: maintaining a healthy diet, using medications, practicing bowel training, and receiving sacral nerve stimulation.
- Total incontinence occurs when there is a complete loss of bladder control.

If you are diagnosed with stress incontinence, even if you feel that your bladder problems are out of control, there are still many non-invasive ways to improve your individual situation. They include using:

- Bladder training.
- Kegel exercises.
- Behavioral and biofeedback therapy.
- Cones and weights.
- Biofeedback devices.
- Mechanical devices.
- Medications.

If a physician recommends surgery, after all other options have been exhausted, examine your alternatives carefully. The various surgical procedures for the different forms of incontinence currently include: bladder neck injections, bladder neck suspension procedures, sling procedures, sacral nerve stimulation, augmentation cystoplasty, and urinary diversion.

We hope we've given you the incentive to confidently deal with any bladder issues you may encounter. Maximizing and improving your continence is well within your reach, no matter your age, health, or other life factors. Go for it. You have nothing to lose, everything to gain, and a wonderful, carefree, liberated life to lead. We wish you the very best of health. Be well.

Appendix I

Incontinence Products

The following products are available for the treatment and management of urinary and fecal incontinence:

Disposable absorbent products

- Intravaginal devices such as Poise Impressa

The disposable panty liners, pads, and panties that are currently available provide excellent protection because:

- New "hook and loop" technology provides for a better fit than the original adhesive closure garments.
- They are more secure and provide better coverage.
- They are curved and contoured like undergarments. They are discreet and natural looking under clothing.
- They are less bulky, yet have greater absorbency.
- They are made from odor-controlling material.
- Some products allow toileting without removal of the entire garment.

Reusable Absorbent Products

Some wearers feel that, cost concerns aside, reusable absorbent products provide a better fit, are more comfortable, and are easier to deal with. Reusables require the wearer to change them, or their disposable inserts, frequently to avoid skin rash, redness, and irritation. Reusable absorbent products include:

- Absorbent pads
- Waterproof undergarments
- Mattress pads, protectors, and covers

Toileting Accessories and Aids

For those whose mobility is limited and who are unable to remove their clothing or reach the toilet in time to avoid an accident, the following products are available:

- Bedside commodes
- The DuraGlide adjustable level glide bath/commode transfer system
- Female urinals

Briefs with a nighttime bed-wetting alarm for adult nighttime incontinence.

Skin Care, Odor Control, and Surface Support Products

- Select products that protect the skin, are easy to use, and that are cost effective. It is important not only to clean the skin, but also to moisturize it and provide a protective ointment barrier as well. Soft, disposable washcloths are available.
- Urine or stool can be deodorized by giving the patient an oral tablet that will significantly reduce or eliminate unpleasant odors associated with urinary and fecal incontinence.
- Pressure-reducing mattresses and chair cushions are available for bedridden or chair-bound individuals. These products provide even weight distribution to avoid skin problems.

Intermittent Self-Catheterization Devices

- A wide variety of catheters are available for women. Some are pre-lubricated.

Pelvic Muscle Training and Rehabilitation Aids and Therapies:
- Biofeedback measuring and monitoring machines
- Strengthening machines
- Combination products

Pessaries
- A wide variety of pessaries are available to support the vagina and the urethra to prevent incontinence. A pessary requires a custom fit.

Medications (See chapter 11)

Appendix II

Bladder Lingo—
A Glossary of Terms

Alzheimer's is a neurologic condition in which memory, speech, muscles, and the intellect progressively deteriorate until the patient can no longer take care of her personal needs.

An **anal electromyography** tests for nerve damage associated with an injury sustained while giving birth.

An **anal manometry** checks the pressure of the rectum when it is resting or when it is squeezing and the sensitivity, capacity, and compliance of the rectum.

Anorectal nerves regulate the sensation and strength of the rectal and anal sphincter muscles.

An **anorectal ultrasound** diagnostic imaging study allows the doctor to evaluate both the internal and external sphincters at work.

Anticholinergic drugs, used for urge incontinence, block the impulses between the nerves that control the bladder and the bladder muscle itself. The response of muscle to stimulation is chemically suppressed. These drugs stop or delay muscle spasms.

An **atonic bladder** is one that doesn't contract or empty properly, possibly due to nerve damage. The bladder fills until it overflows with excess urine that dribbles out.

Atrophic vaginitis is a condition in which the vagina becomes inflamed due to tissues that shrink and become thin as a result of decreased lubrication of the vaginal walls. This condition is caused by the lack of estrogen normally associated with menopause.

Augmentation cystoplasty is a major operation performed for severe urge incontinence or urinary frequency only when all other non-invasive procedures and treatments have proven ineffective. This surgery involves taking a piece of the intestine and using it to reconstruct the bladder by enlarging it to increase its capacity.

Behavioral therapy focuses on retraining the brain to control the bladder more effectively and efficiently by suppressing involuntary bladder contractions.

Biofeedback devices provide pelvic floor muscle stimulation, which allows the user to have increased voluntary control over urine storage.

A **bladder diary** records fluid intake and the frequency, timing, and volume of voids, as well as the number and severity of incontinent episodes and the activity associated with the event.

Bladder instability is another term for urge incontinence.

Bladder instillation is a type of bladder wash or bath used to relieve symptoms of interstitial cystitis.

The **bladder** is a hollow, muscle-lined sac located in the lower abdomen that stores urine and then later eliminates it.

The **bladder neck** is an area at the base of the bladder where it connects to the top of the urethra.

Bladder neck injections of collagen or other synthetic bulking agents are placed in the wall of the urethra to strengthen it so that urine can't leak out as easily.

Bladder neck suspension surgery is performed to stabilize the support for the urethra and the bladder.

BMI stands for "body mass index," a numerical value of your weight in relation to your height.

"Camel bladder" occurs in certain women who void infrequently, have a large-capacity bladder, and yet show no evidence of urethral obstruction or an impaired detrusor muscle. Over time, this may lead to voiding difficulties.

Catheterization is the act of inserting a catheter to relieve urine retention.

A **catheter** is a long, thin tube inserted into the bladder to allow the urine to drain from the bladder.

The **cervix** is the lowest part of the uterus (which dilates during labor) and extends into and is attached to the vagina.

Chronic incontinence develops slowly over a considerable amount of time and results from damage to or abnormalities in muscles and nerves, or from gradual changes to the bladder or urethra.

Coital incontinence refers to the leaking of urine during sexual intercourse.

Collagen is a connective tissue protein substance in the skin that supports it. It is also a common substance found in animal bones and connective tissue. Bovine cross-linked GAX collagen is taken from cattle, purified, and then readied for use in humans.

A **colostomy (ileostomy)** involves removing a portion of the bowel and attaching the remaining portion either to the anus (if it works properly) or to a hole in the abdomen called a stoma, through which stool leaves the body and is collected in a special bag.

Cystitis is an inflammation of the bladder that is most commonly caused by a bacterial infection and most effectively treated with antibiotics.

A **cystocele** occurs when the bladder drops down into the vagina, which may result in incomplete emptying of the bladder and, possibly, urinary tract infections. A cystocele may become worse with time, age, and gravity.

A **cystometer** is the machine that performs a cystometry. Another term for this is a urodynamics machine.

A **cystometrogram (CMG)** graph measures the capacity, irritability, and elasticity of the bladder.

Cystometry is the measurement of the pressure and volume of the bladder both when full and when empty.

A **cystoscope** is a thin, narrow telescope passed through the urethra into the bladder allowing the doctor look inside that organ.

Cystoscopy is a procedure used to diagnose urinary tract disorders whereby a rigid or flexible, thin, telescope-like instrument is inserted first into the urethra and then into the bladder, allowing for a direct view of both.

Defecography (See proctography)

Dementia, or gradual mental deterioration, is a condition wherein the patient loses her memory, her language and problem solving skills, her ability to learn, her judgment, and her ability to perform daily activities.

Detrusor hyperreflexia occurs when there is a neurological cause for involuntary bladder contractions. Spasms result from damage to the nerves of the bladder, nervous system, or the bladder muscles themselves.

Detrusor instability is another term for urge incontinence. It refers to an unstable bladder, one in which the detrusor muscle (the muscle responsible for contracting the bladder so that urine can be voided) contracts involuntarily and for no apparent reason.

The **detrusor muscle** makes up the entire outside of the bladder and is responsible for contracting the bladder during urination.

Detrusor overactivity is characterized by involuntary detrusor contractions during the filling phase.

Diabetes is a disease wherein an individual has an abnormal blood sugar level due to a lack of insulin, a substance produced in the pancreas. When the blood sugar level increases, great thirst occurs, and urinary frequency can become an outcome.

Diabetic cystopathy occurs when the myelin sheath surrounding the bladder nerves becomes damaged. This causes communication problems between the brain and the bladder and prevents the bladder and the sphincter from functioning normally.

Dysuria is pain or difficulty in urinating commonly caused by inflammation or infection.

Ectopic ureter is one that is not in its correct place: it may not connect to the bladder but enter the urethra or the vagina instead.

An **electromyogram** (EMG) evaluates whether the pelvic muscles are contracting and relaxing properly.

An **enterocele** occurs when the small intestine drops into the vagina. It is seen as a bulge and is covered with vaginal epithelium or skin.

An **episiotomy** is an incision made during childbirth to the perineum, the muscle between the vagina and rectum, to enlarge the vaginal opening, thus making it easier for the baby to emerge. It reduces the likelihood that the pelvic muscles will tear irregularly.

Eyeball urodynamics (a.k.a. "bedside cystometrics") is used to obtain diagnostic information about the bladder without using electronic equipment.

Fecal incontinence refers to the inability to control one's bowels voluntarily, causing stool, liquid, or gas to leak unexpectedly and uncontrollably from the rectum.

A **fistula** is a hole from one organ to another. A bladder fistula is a hole in the bladder causing leaking from the bladder into the urethra or the vagina.

A **flowmeter** measures the quantity of fluid in cubic centimeters voided per unit of times (usually per second).

A **Foley (indwelling) catheter** is a long-term use catheter for a person with urinary incontinence or retention that cannot be treated with medication, surgery, or self-intermittent catheterization.

With **functional incontinence**, there is not a problem with bladder function and control per se, but an inability or unwillingness on the part of the individual to reach a bathroom in time due to loss of mobility.

Glycosaminoglycan (GAG) is a layer of protein that lines and shields the bladder from the invasion of toxins and chemicals.

A **gracilis muscle transplant (graciloplasty)** is performed to restore muscle tone to the sphincter and involves replacing the anal sphincter muscle with muscle from the patient's inner thigh.

Hematuria is blood in the urine.

A **hemorrhoid** is an enlarged vein in the rectum or anus.

Hemorrhoidectomy is surgery to remove a hemorrhoid and any underlying problems.

Hesitancy occurs when the individual can't get the urine stream started despite every effort.

Homeostasis refers to the balance of the body's internal environment, e.g., blood pressure, temperature, blood sugar level.

A **hyposensitive** bladder is generally due to reduced nerve sensation that causes a person to lose the desire to urinate.

Idiopathic refers to a disease of unknown origin.

Ileostomy (See colostomy)

Impressa is a disposable, tampon-like device that treats stress incontinence. It is inserted inside the vagina and can be used for up to eight hours at a time.

Indwelling catheter (See Foley catheter)

Intermittency occurs when the urine flow stops and starts, following an "on-off" pattern that causes the individual to drip or dribble and feel that the bladder hasn't been completely emptied even though only an insignificant amount of urine may be retained.

Interstitial cystitis is a condition typified by chronic inflammation, thickening, and scarring of the bladder lining that causes frequency and urgency and can cause the bladder lining to bleed into the urine.

An **intravenous urogram** examines the anatomy of the kidneys, ureters, and bladder.

Irritable bladder is another term for urge incontinence.

Kegel pelvic muscle exercises help tremendously with bladder control by strengthening and retraining the pelvic muscles and by improving the strength and timing of pelvic floor muscle contractions.

The **kidneys** constantly filter the body's blood supply by separating and eliminating toxins and waste products from those elements that the body needs in order to maintain homeostasis.

Laparoscopy is a procedure where the surgeon uses a small video camera and a few specialized instruments to perform surgery with minimal incisions.

Micturition reflex refers to the entire process of urination: the relaxation of the sphincter muscles, the contraction of the bladder, the relaxation and opening of the urethra, and the act of voiding.

Mixed incontinence is generally a combination of stress and urge incontinence. This usually requires a urodynamic workup for a proper diagnosis.

Motor urgency occurs when the detrusor muscle is unstable and causes involuntary contractions, leakage, or the immediate release of urine, creating a gushing feeling.

Multiple sclerosis is a chronic, debilitating, degenerative disease of the nervous system.

Myelin is a fatty protein that encases nerves. The myelin sheath is responsible for the proper transmission of nerve impulses.

A **neurogenic** bladder malfunctions due to damaged nerves associated with a neurological condition.

Nocturia refers to being awakened during the night by the urge to urinate.

Overflow incontinence occurs when an individual cannot fully empty her bladder when she urinates. This causes too much urine to collect in the bladder and its eventual overflow (because it is full), resulting in involuntary leakage or dribbling.

A **pad test** determines the amount of urine leakage.

Parkinson's disease is a slowly progressing, degenerative neurologic disease of the nervous system characterized by tremors, rigidity, a shuffling gait, and bladder problems.

A **pelvic block** maneuver is done by contracting the pelvic floor quickly and tightly prior to a cough, sneeze, or any action that usually results in incontinence.

Pelvic floor muscles are strong, flexible, voluntary skeletal muscles that are attached to the pubic bone and to the tailbone (coccyx). They act as a sling to support and anchor the organs they surround within the abdomen: the uterus, the bladder, and the rectum.

Percutaneous Tibial Nerve Stimulation (PTNS) is an outpatient treatment option for patients with overactive bladder. It involves inserting a small, acupuncture-like electrode on the inner side of the ankle.

The **perineal region** is the area between the vagina and the rectum.

Peristalsis refers to waves of muscular contractions that can occur in the ureter as well as in other organs of the body.

A **pessary** is a nonsurgical, mechanical device that is inserted into the vagina to ensure the support of the pelvic organs in cases of prolapse.

Polyuria refers to the excessive excretion of urine at night.

The **postvoid residual urine volume (PVR)** is the amount of urine that remains in your bladder after you've voided. A PVR of more than 150–200 cc of urine usually indicates a problem.

Procidentia refers to the most severe form of prolapse, where the vagina and uterus sag to a point where they are outside the body.

A **proctography**, also known as a defecography, shows the capacity of the rectum, how well it holds stool, and how well it can evacuate the stool.

A **proctosigmoidoscopy** allows a doctor to look inside your rectum for signs of diseases or tumors, inflammation, or scar tissue that may be responsible for fecal incontinence.

Prolapse is the protrusion, dropping, or sagging of pelvic organs (uterus, bladder, rectum, and small intestine) into the vagina.

Pubovaginal sling surgery is performed to correct types of stress incontinence. In this procedure, a sling is placed around the urethra to provide support during stressful physical activities and also at rest.

The **pudendal** nerve controls the muscles of the pelvic floor, which surround the birth canal.

A **Q-Tip** or cotton swab test determines the type of incontinence.

Quick flick Kegels are performed so that the pelvic muscles are eventually able to tighten and relax as quickly as possible under conditions of physical stress in order to prevent leakage.

Reflex incontinence is the result of involuntary bladder contractions that occur when the urge to urinate is completely absent.

A **rectocele** occurs when the rectum protrudes into the vagina, which may result in incomplete rectal emptying.

The **sacral nerve** runs from the lower spinal cord to the bladder and is responsible for stimulating the muscles and organs involved in bladder control and pelvic floor contractions.

Self-intermittent catheterization is the insertion of a catheter by the patient to alleviate symptoms of bladder retention.

Sensory urgency is when the bladder feels very uncomfortably full but when there is no actual leakage of urine.

A **sonogram** uses ultrasonic wave technology in order to view the kidneys, bladder, and other pelvic organs.

A **sphincter** is a muscle which surrounds a body opening (the urethra or the anus, for example) and which should unconsciously remain tightly closed.

Sphincter incompetence (urethral) is another way of referring to stress urinary incontinence.

Sphincteroplasty is surgery to repair a damaged or weakened anal sphincter.

Spina bifida is a birth defect caused by the failure of the fetus's spine to close properly during the first month of pregnancy. Although the spinal opening can be surgically repaired shortly after birth, the nerve damage is permanent, resulting in varying degrees of paralysis of the lower limbs as well as bladder and bowel problems. The individual may not feel the urge to urinate when the bladder contracts, which results in incontinence.

Stress incontinence refers to involuntary leakage of urine due to lack of sufficient urethral closure pressure.

Stress tests check for the loss of urine.

Stroke victims initially experience urinary frequency, urgency, and urge incontinence caused by involuntary bladder contractions.

Sympathomimetic drugs, used for stress incontinence, tighten the muscles at the bladder neck. They cannot be taken with most drugs for Parkinson's disease or with drugs for high pressure. They may cause hypertensive reactions, headache, nausea, vomiting, and palpitations.

Total incontinence refers to a complete loss of bladder control.

Transient incontinence is usually caused by an illness or a specific medical condition that is more or less short-lived and is, therefore, quickly remedied by appropriate treatment of the condition and disappearance of symptoms.

Ultrasound (See sonogram)

An **underactive detrusor** muscle doesn't provide the necessary stimulation for the bladder to contract properly in order to eliminate enough urine.

An **unstable bladder** is another term for urge incontinence.

Ureters are narrow, hollow, muscular tubes, approximately nine inches long, which connect each kidney to the bladder.

Urethral incompetence is another way of referring to the ISD form of stress urinary incontinence.

The **urethra**, located above the vaginal opening, is the short (three to four centimeter), narrow tube that carries urine from the bladder to the outside of the body.

Urethral hypermobility refers to too much movement of the urethra, causing it to drop below the pelvic floor muscles during certain activities, which may cause leakage.

Urethritis is an inflammation of the urethra.

A **urethroscopy** checks that the bladder, the uterus, the vagina, and the rectum are anatomically correct.

Urge incontinence refers to the sensation that urination is imminent and that it cannot be postponed for more than a few seconds or minutes, resulting in leakage of urine.

Urinary diversion is surgery that is performed when the bladder and/or urethra are damaged beyond repair and no longer serve a useful function. Urine is diverted to a urinary reservoir that serves as a new bladder or to a urinary conduit that allows the individual to pass urine through a stoma in the abdomen into a drainage bag.

Urinary incontinence (UI), as defined by the International Continence Society, is "involuntary urine loss that is sufficient to be a social or hygienic problem and is objectively demonstrable."

Urinary retention is when a person cannot urinate. Retention is caused by a urethral blockage or impaired bladder contractions.

The **urinary tract** is the passageway through which bodily waste products are filtered and through which urine is produced, stored, and excreted. A urinalysis and culture checks for infection, inflammation, crystals, protein, blood, and/or sugar (glucose) in the urine.

Urodynamic testing is a sophisticated way to reproduce bladder symptoms and to pinpoint specific problems in order to evaluate bladder function.

Urodynamics is the study of and a series of tests determining how the bladder, urethra, and pelvic floor muscles function.

Uroflowmetry tests for blockages in the urethra and abnormal voiding patterns, and measures the strength, volume, and smoothness of urinary flow and how long it takes to urinate and to stop urinating.

Urogynecologists are doctors with specialized training in feminine urologic and gynecologic problems. They examine and treat conditions that affect the muscles and tissues that support female pelvic organs.

Urologists are doctors with specialized training in the urinary tract.

Uterine prolapse occurs when the uterus and cervix drop down into the vagina.

UTI stands for urinary tract infection.

Vaginal cones are used to strengthen pelvic muscles and reduce unwanted bladder contractions.

Vaginitis is a condition in which the vaginal walls become thin and the vagina becomes irritated and inflamed, causing soreness and itching.

Valsalva leak point pressure (VLPP) is used to measure the competency of the urethra.

Appendix III

Organizations and Websites
That Really Help

For help with urinary and fecal incontinence, visit the websites or call the organizations listed below:

Alzheimer's Disease and Related Disorders
Phone: (800) 272-3900
www.alz.org

American Cancer Society, Inc.
Phone: (800) ACS (227)-2345
www.cancer.org

The American College of Obstetricians and Gynecologists (ACOG)
Phone: (800) 673-8444
www.acog.org

American Diabetes Association
Phone: (800) 342-2383
www.diabetes.org

American Kidney Fund
Phone: (888) 560-8232
www.kidneyfund.org

American Parkinson Disease Association, Inc.
Phone: (800) 223-2732
www.apdaparkinson.org

American Physical Therapy Association (APTA)
Phone: (800) 999-2782
www.apta.org

American Society on Aging
Phone: (800) 537-9728
www.asaging.org

The American Urologic Association (AUA
Phone (410) 689-3700
www.AUAnet.org

Crohn's & Colitis Foundation of America, Inc.
Phone: (800) 932-2423
www.crohnscolitisfoundation.org

IC Network
Phone: (707) 538-9442
www.ic-network.com

Interstitial Cystitis Association of America (ICA)
Phone: (800) 928-7496
www.ichelp.org

Michael J. Fox Foundation
Phone: (800) 708-7644
michaeljfox.org

Multiple Sclerosis Association of America (MSAA)
Phone: (800) 532-7667
www.msaa.com

National Association for Continence
Phone: (800) BLADDER (252-3337)
www.nafc.org

National Council on Aging (NCOA)
Phone: (571) 527-3900
www.ncoa.org

National Health Information Center (NHIC)
www.health.gov/nhic

National Kidney and Urologic Diseases Information Clearinghouse
(NKUDIC)
www.kidney.niddk.nih.gov/kudiseases/pubs/bladdercontrol/in-
dex.htm

National Kidney Foundation
Phone: (877) 963-7033
www.kidney.org

National Multiple Sclerosis Society (NMSS)
Phone: (800) 344-4867
www.nmss.org

National Spinal Cord Injury Association (NSCIA)
Phone: (800) 913-6370
www.spinal-cord.org

National Stroke Association (NSA)
www.stroke.org

The Simon Foundation for Continence
Phone: (800) 237-4666
www.simonfoundation.org

Society for Women's Health Research (SWHR)
Phone: (202) 223-8244
www.swhr.org

Spina Bifida Association of America (SPAA)
Phone: (800) 621-3141
www.sbaa.org

United Ostomy Association
Phone: (800) 826-0826
www.ostomy.org

United Spinal Association
Phone: (718) 803-3782
www.unitedspinal.org

Should you find other websites on your own, use these guidelines to determine whether they are credible and reliable. Remember, the internet is a valuable tool, but it does not take the place of qualified, personalized medical care.

- The owner and purpose of the website should be clearly indicated. Any advertisers, sponsors, or funding should be noted so that you can determine who has a personal interest in the site.
- The material should be written or reviewed by qualified healthcare providers. Websites written by government agencies or by national medical associations can be trusted to provide accurate and reliable information.
- The website should provide its privacy policy to let you know how your rights are protected.
- Health websites should list all references (articles, books, etc.) used to obtain the information provided. These materials should be current.
- Medical information often changes and should be regularly updated. Health websites should provide the date of the last update so you can ascertain whether you think the information is recent enough to suit your needs.[84]

Bibliography

Abrams P, Cardozo L, Fall M, et al. 2002. The standardization of terminology of lower urinary tract function: report from the standardization sub-committee of the International Continence Society. Am J Obstet Gynecol 187:116–26.

Abrams P, Cardozo L, Fall M., et al. 2002. The standardization of terminology of lower urinary tract function: report from the standardization sub-committee of the International Continence Society. Am J Obstet Gynecol 187:116–26.

American College of Physicians. 2000. Urinary Incontinence in Women. London: Dorling Kindersley.

American Urogynecologic Society (AUGS) website. Available from: www.augs.org

Bo K, Talseth T.. 1996. Long-term effect of pelvic floor muscle exercise 5 years after cessation of organized training. Obstet Gynecol 87:378–9.

Brown JS, Sawaya G, Thom D, Grady D, Lancet. 2000. Hysterectomy and urinary incontinence: a systematic review. JAMA. 356:535–539

Burgio KL, Locher JL, Goode PS, et al. 1998. Behavioral vs drug treatment for urge urinary incontinence in older women: a randomized controlled trial. JAMA 280:1995–2000.

Carrington, E. V., Scott, S. M., Bharucha, A., Mion, F., Remes-Troche, J. M., Malcolm, A., & Rao, S. S. (2018). Expert consensus document: advances in the evaluation of anorectal function. Nature Reviews Gastroenterology & Hepatology/ 15(5): 309.

Cheung, O., & Wald, A. (2004). The management of pelvic floor disorders. Alimentary pharmacology & therapeutics. 19(5): 481-495.

Choe JM. Pubovaginal Sling. eMedicine.

Conquering Bladder and Prostate Problems, The Authoritative Guide for Men and Women. Blaivas JG. New York: Perseus Press, 2001. ...

Culligan PJ, Heit M. Urinary incontinence in women: evaluation and management. Am Fam Phys 2000 Dec 1; 62(11):2433–2444, 2447, 2452.

Del Río-Gonzalez, S., Aragon, I. M., Castillo, E., Milla-España, F., Galacho, A., Machuca, J., ... & Herrera-Imbroda, B. (2017). Percutaneous tibial nerve stimulation therapy for overactive bladder syndrome: clinical effectiveness, urodynamic, and durability evaluation. Urology. 108: 52-58.

Diokno A, Brock B, Brown M, Herzog A. 1986. Prevalence of urinary incontinence and other urological symptoms in the noninstitutionalized elderly. J Urol 136:1022–5.

Fantl JA, et al. 1996. Urinary Incontinence in Adults: Acute and Chronic Management. NIDDK [Internet]. (Development of a computer-based system for continence health promotion. Nursing Outlook, Volume 52, Issue 5, Pages 241-247 A. Boyington, B. Wildemuth, M. Dougherty, E. Palenahall)

Gleason, J. L., Richter, H. E., Redden, D. T., Goode, P. S., Burgio, K. L., & Markland, A. D. (2013). Caffeine and urinary incontinence in US women. International urogynecology journal.24(2): 295-302.

Gormley, E. A., Lightner, D. J., Faraday, M., & Vasavada, S. P. (2015). Diagnosis and treatment of overactive bladder (non-neurogenic) in adults: AUA/SUFU guideline amendment. The Journal of urology. 193(5): 1572-1580

Gray, T., Li, W., Campbell, P., Jha, S., & Radley, S. (2018). Evaluation of coital incontinence by electronic questionnaire: prevalence, associations and outcomes in women attending a urogynaecology clinic. International urogynecology journal. 29(7): 969-978.

Handavl GH, Gold E, Robbins J. 2004. Progression and remission of pelvic organ prolapse—a longitudinal study of menopausal women. Am J Obstet Gynecol 190(1):27–32

Hay-Smith EJ, et al. 2001. Cochrane Database Syst Rev 1: CD001407.

Hendrix, S. L., Cochrane, B. B., Nygaard, I. E., Handa, V. L., Barnabei, V. M., Iglesia, C., ... & McNeeley, S. G. (2005). Effects of estrogen with and without progestin on urinary incontinence. Jama. 293(8): 935-948.

Hu TW, Impact of urinary incontinence on healthcare costs. 2004, Journal of the American Geriatrics Society 38(3):292–295.

Jackson SL, Weber AM, Hull TL, Mitchinson AR, Walters MD. 1997. Fecal incontinence in women with urinary incontinence and pelvic organ prolapse. Obstet Gynecol 89(3):423–7.
JAMA. May 12, 1989. 261(18).

Johanson JF, Lafferty J. Jan., 1996. Epidemiology of fecal incontinence: the silent affliction. Am J Gastroenterol 91(1):33–6. [Medline].

Kalant H, Grant D, Mitchell J. 2006. Principles of Medical Pharmacology, Seventh ed. Part 2, Autonomic Nervous System. Saunders, Toronto, Canada.

Levy, R, Muller, N. Urinary Incontinence: Economic Burden and New Choices in Pharmaceutical Treatment. Advances in Therapy, Vol 23, No 4, July/August 2006.

Li Y, Cai X, Glance LG, Mukamel DB. Nov., 2007. Gender differences in healthcare-seeking behavior for urinary incontinence and the impact of socioeconomic status: a study of the Medicare managed care population. Med Care 45(11):1116–22.

Lukban JC, et al. 2006. Int Urolgynecol J [Internet].

M. Nawal Lutfiyya[1], Deepa K. Bhat[2], Seema R. Gandhi[3], Catherine Nguyen[4], Vicki L. Weidenbacher-Hoper[1] and Martin S. Lipsky[1] A comparison of quality of care indicators in urban acute care hospitals and rural critical access hospitals in the United States. International Journal for Quality in Health Care 2007 19(3):141-149

Mardon, RE, Halim, S, et al 2005. Management of Urinary Incontinence in Medicare Managed Care Beneficiaries. Journal of the American Medical Association. March 2005. 293(8):935–948.

NAFC. Quality Care 20(1).

NAFC. Your Personal Guide to Bladder Health. [Updated July, 2007].

National Kidney and Urologic Diseases Information Clearinghouse, NIH. July, 2007.

Nelson R, Norton N, Cautley E, Furner S. Aug. 16, 1995. Community-based prevalence of anal incontinence. JAMA: 274(7):559–61 [Medline].

Newman DK. 1999. The Urinary Incontinence Sourcebook. New York: McGraw Hill Education.

Nygaard, C. C., Schreiner, L., Morsch, T. P., Saadi, R. P., Figueiredo, M. F., & Padoin, A. V. (2019). Urinary Incontinence and Surgery for Obesity and Weight-Related Diseases: Are There Predictors of Improvement?. Obesity surgery. 29(1): 109-113.

Nygaard I, Cruickshank D. 2003. Should all women be offered elective caesarean delivery? Obstet and Gynecol 102: 217–219.

Nygaard IE, Thompson FL, Svengalis SL, Albright JP. 1994. Urinary incontinence in elite nulliparous athletes. Obstet Gyn 84:183–187.

Nygaard, et al. Is urinary incontinence a barrier to exercise in women? 2005. Obstet Gynecol 106(2):307.

O'Donnel PD. Urinary incontinence in America: the social significance. 2002. St. Louis (MO): Mosby Yearbook Inc. .

Olsen AL, Smith VJ, Bergstrom JO, Colling JC, Clark AL. 1997. Epidemiology of surgically managed pelvic organ prolapse and urinary incontinence. Obstet Gynecol 89:501–6.

Rabin JM, Stern JR. 2002. You're Never Too Old To Have Fun—Tips on Staying Young and Being Healthy. New York: Stern/Greco Publishers. p 17.

Rinne KM, Kirkinem PP. 1999. What predisposes young women to genital prolapse? EUR J Obstet Gynecol Reprod Biol 84:23–5.

Robinson, D., & Cardozo, L. D. (2003). The role of estrogens in female lower urinary tract dysfunction. Urology.62(4): 45-51.

Rohner TJ, Rohner JF. 1997. Urinary Incontinence in America: The social significance. In P. D. O'Donnel (ed.), Urinary Incontinence. St. Louis (MO):Mosby Yearbook.

Seymour SD. emedicine [Internet].

Subak LL, Quesenberry CP, Posner SF, Cattolica E, Soghikian K. 2002. The effect of behavioral therapy on urinary incontinence: a randomized controlled trial. Obstet Gynecol 100:72–8.

Swenson, C. (2018). Urinary Incontinence: An Inevitable Part of Aging?

Swithinbank L, Hashim H, Abrams P. The effect of fluid intake on urinary symptoms in women. The Journal of Urology 174(1):187– 189

Urinary Incontinence Guideline Panel. March, 1992. Urinary incontinence in adults: clinical practice guidelines. Agency for Healthcare Policy and Research, Public Health Service. Rockville (MD): U.S. Department of Health and Human Services.

Urinary Incontinence in Adults: Clinical Practice Guideline. AHCPR Pub. No. 92-0038. Rockville, MD: Agency for Healthcare Policy and Research, Public Health Service, U.S. Department of Health and Human Services. March, 1992. Also cited from Thomas TM, Plymat KR, Blannin J, & Meade TW. 1980. Prevalence of urinary incontinence. British Medical J 281(6250):1243–1245.

Wagner. 1998. Economic Considerations of Overactive Bladder. Urology 51(3)355–361.

Wall LE, Davidson TG. 1992. The role of muscular re-education by physical therapists in the diagnosis of genuine stress urinary incontinence. Obstet Gynecol Surg 47: 322–31.

Weber, A, Walters, M. et al. Sexual function in women with uterovaginal prolapse and urinary incontinence. Obstet Gynecol. 1995; 85: 483–487.

Wesnes, S. L., Rortveit, G., Bø, K., & Hunskaar, S. (2007). Urinary incontinence during pregnancy. Obstetrics & Gynecology. 109(4): 922-928

"What is incontinence?" National Association for Continence website. 2006. Available from: www.nafc.org

www.fascrs.org/patients/disease-condition/fecal-incontinence-0

www.grandviewresearch.com/industry-analysis/adult-diapers-market

www.healthline.com/health/multiple-sclerosis/facts-statistics-infographic#1.

www.hemorrhoid.net/fecalincon.php

www.ichelp.org/about-ic/what-is-interstitial-cystitis/4-to-12-million-may-have-ic.

www.managedhealthcareconnect.com/article/5554

www.mayoclinic.com. Fecal Incontinence.

www.mayoclinic.com. Interstitial cystitis. Treatment.

www.mayoclinic.com. Multiple sclerosis. Overview. Signs and symptoms.

www.urologychannel.com.interstitialcystitis/index.shtml

www.yourpelvicfloor.org

Xu, X., Menees, S. B., Zochowski, M. K., & Fenner, D. E. (2012). Economic cost of fecal incontinence. Diseases of the Colon & Rectum, 55(5), 586-598.

About the Authors

Dr. Jill M. Rabin, an award-winning physician, is a Professor of Obstetrics and Gynecology at the Zucker School of Medicine at Hofstra Northwell, Vice Chair for Education and Development at North Shore University Hospital and LIJ Medical Center/Northwell Health, Co-Chief of Ambulatory Care in OBGYN/Northwell Health, and Section Head of Urogynecology at LIJ/Northwell.

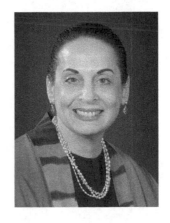

Dr. Rabin, a Diplomate of the American Board of Obstetrics and Gynecology, is an active researcher, consultant, lecturer, and media spokesperson. She holds eight patents and one copyright for urogynecologic medical devices, including a confidence-building incontinence pad, a pessary for treating vaginal prolapse, and a finger protector for surgeons. In recognition of her professional excellence, she has garnered many research and teaching awards, including the excellence in teaching award from the Association of Professors in Gynecology and Obstetrics. Widely published, she has authored four books on women's health.

As a physician, Dr. Rabin is passionate about improving the lives of women by providing them with quality healthcare and up-to-the-minute medical information. As a teacher, she is dedicated to enhancing and enriching the medical education of her students through progressive curriculum development and active mentorship. It is her firm belief that empowered patients and compassionate, well-prepared physicians can work together to greatly improve women's health.

Gail Stein, M.A. is a retired New York City junior and senior high school foreign language instructor. During her more than thirty-three years of service she assisted in a revision project of the French curriculum for the New York City Board of Education, served as an adjunct professor to St. John's University in its Early Admission Extension Program, gave presentations and demonstrations at numerous citywide foreign language conferences, appeared on the Barry Farber radio program

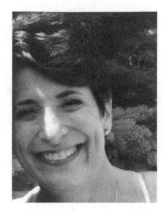

promoting the study of French, and had her lessons videotaped by the New York City Board of Education for national distribution. Mrs. Stein is a multiple-time honoree in *Who's Who Among America's Teachers*.

In addition to *Mind Over Bladder*, Gail Stein is the author of over forty well-known French and Spanish textbooks, phrase books, guides, handbooks, and a crossword puzzle book.

Mrs. Stein is a longtime patient and friend of Dr. Jill M. Rabin.

Danielle O'Shaughnessy, MD, FACOG is a practicing Urogynecologist in Eastern Long Island. Dr. O'Shaughnessy earned her MD from the State University of New York, Downstate Medical Center, in Brooklyn. She then completed a residency in Obstetrics and Gynecology at Northwell Health System, and continued in the Northwell Health System to complete a fellowship in Female Pelvic Medicine and Reconstructive Surgery. After fellowship, she joined Northwell Physician Partners.

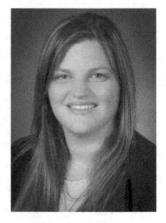

Her research interested include optimizing a surgical graft material for use in prolapse and incontinence. She currently serves as the Research Director for the Female Pelvic Medicine and Reconstructive Surgery Fellowship at Northwell Health as well as Assistant Professor in Department of OB/GYN Donald and Zucker School of Medicine at Hofstra/Northwell. Dr. O'Shaughnessy is a member of several professional organizations, including the American Urogynecologic Society and American Board of Obstetrics and Gynecology.